More Cognitively Advanced Individuals with *Autism Spectrum Disorders*

by the same author

The Partner's Guide to Asperger Syndrome
Susan J. Moreno, Marci Wheeler and Kealah Parkinson
Foreword by Tony Attwood
ISBN 978 1 84905 878 0
eISBN 978 0 85700 566 3

of related interest

Raising Children with Asperger's Syndrome and High-functioning Autism
Championing the Individual
Yuko Yoshida MD
Illustrated by Jun'ichi Sato
Translated by Esther Sanders and Cathy Hirano
ISBN 978 1 84905 317 4
eISBN 978 0 85700 660 8

The Complete Guide to Asperger's Syndrome
Tony Attwood
ISBN 978 1 84310 495 7 (hardback)
ISBN 978 1 84310 669 2 (paperback)
eISBN 978 1 84642 559 2

More Cognitively Advanced Individuals with *Autism Spectrum Disorders*

Autism, Asperger Syndrome and PDD/NOS—the Basics

Susan J. Moreno, MAABS

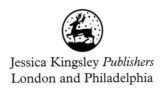

Jessica Kingsley *Publishers*
London and Philadelphia

Appendix B reproduced from Moreno 1992 with kind permission from Gary Mesibov and Springer Science+Business Media B.V.

First published in 2013
by Jessica Kingsley Publishers
116 Pentonville Road
London N1 9JB, UK
and
400 Market Street, Suite 400
Philadelphia, PA 19106, USA

www.jkp.com

Library of Congress Cataloging in Publication Data
Moreno, Susan.
    More cognitively advanced individuals with autism spectrum disorders : autism, asperger syndrome and PDD/NOS-- the basics / Susan J. Moreno ; foreword by Susan J. Moreno. -- 2nd ed.
       p. cm.
    Includes bibliographical references and index.
    ISBN 978-1-84905-910-7 (alk. paper)
    1. Autism spectrum disorders--Popular works. I. Title.
    RC553.A88M678 2012
    616.85'882--dc23
                                        2012020910

British Library Cataloguing in Publication Data
A CIP catalogue record for this book is available from the British Library

ISBN 978 1 84905 910 7
eISBN 978 0 85700 699 8

Printed and bound in the United States

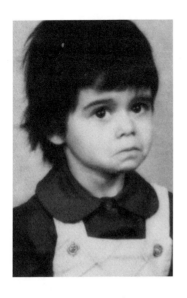 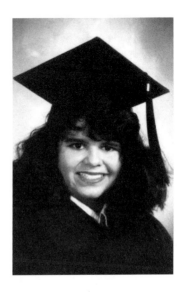

How did we get from here...   to here?

Contents

Preface

This book is a revision of my previous work *High Functioning Individuals with Autism*. The sales and feedback on that book have been tremendous. However, some of the information needed to be updated. Since the writing of the original work, I have been further educated—by the thousands of new parents and more advanced individuals (see Glossary) I have met, by absorbing new research and information, and most importantly by my wonderful daughter Beth as she has grown into a young woman.

Again, I want to thank Dr. Anne Donnellan, without whom neither my newsletter nor my booklet would ever have been created in the first place. Additional thanks to Dr. Bennett Leventhal, my mentor and friend of many years, and to Dr. Cathy Pratt, who has kept my ideas and energy up to par and who has assisted me in editing this book and in keeping MAAP Services a thriving and vital organization. Thanks also go to Dr. Gary Mesibov for encouraging me to write down any experiences and regarding me as a professional.

Above all, I thank my family: Marco, Beth and Mandy. Marco, I thank you for being there for me in every way through good times and bad and for being a wonderful father to our girls. I thank God that I found you and that you have graced me with your love. Mandy, I thank you for forgiving me for years of feeling in last place in family priorities. I hope that now you know that those things happened because I thought you were the strongest and didn't realize all of your fears. Despite that, you have been and always will be my sunshine and treasure. Beth, I will never be able to thank you for the lessons you've taught me—not just about autism, but about human courage and spirit. I cherish you and wouldn't have traded the experience of being your mother for all of the riches on earth. I'm so glad we have *fun* together, too.

My hope for other parents who read this is that they will experience the fullness and joy in life we have had because usually we were given the best information possible at the times we needed it. There were many "bumps" along the road to where we are now. Of course, Beth's success is due to hard work: by professionals who helped her and us; by her mother, father and sister; by caring friends, tutors, and coworkers. Mostly, the credit is due to *Beth*. Her energy, determination, and intelligence tipped the balance. But in retrospect, we were also incredibly lucky.

I know many parents and individuals with autism spectrum disorders (ASDs) (see Glossary) who have worked just as hard, or harder, and things have been different for them. Their offspring with an ASD worked just as hard as Beth. They, too, have found success, but sometimes that success is measured differently. Perhaps that success is learning the independence skills to live in a group home or shared apartment. Or it could be that they have shed behaviors that would have prevented them from work and recreational activities that they now enjoy. Beth's success lies in her academic accomplishments (Master's degree) and in using her talents in voice and languages.

I hope this book will help in some small way. I don't claim to be a better parent than anyone who reads this book. I certainly don't claim to have all of the answers! What I do promise is that I will do my best to use clear, non-technical language and be honest in presenting what I've lived and what I've learned.

Introduction

The purpose of this work is to offer information and suggestions about more advanced individuals with autism, Asperger syndrome, and pervasive developmental disorder— not otherwise specified. I include all three of these DSM-IV-TR categories (see Glossary), because I share the belief that they are all parts of the autism spectrum. "More advanced" individuals typically have normal or above intelligence, but suffer the social, communication, and cognitive problems of autism, although in different, less visible ways than more severely challenged individuals with autism. For example, they may want and need friends, but may not have the skills to make and keep close friends, yet they have many "casual friends." They may have highly articulate speech, but may not be effective in understanding what is important in things said to them or may not be able to communicate their problem in an emergency or under stress. Also, they may continue a rigid way of thinking and inflexible adaptations to change. In addition, many exhibit disabilities of learning in some or many academic subjects, despite their intelligence level and areas of above normal skill.

There is a danger that this book or others may unnecessarily emphasize the differences between these individuals and others with autism. These differences may, in fact, be more apparent than real. Nonetheless, the book is needed because the condition of autism in a person who *appears* so capable presents such unusual challenges. It is a non-visible disability, and clear literature on the topic that doesn't promote one specific treatment and is written in non-technical language is still very scarce.

My knowledge on this subject is drawn primarily from my experiences as the parent of a daughter in her adult years who, in addition to being a talented singer, a music minister in her church, fluent in three languages, and a college graduate with a master's degree, has autism. Our family's success and good fortune in helping Beth cope with and overcome many of her symptomatic behaviors has prompted me to work as an advisor to other families of more advanced individuals. I do this through my work at MAAP Services and our quarterly newsletter, *The MAAP Newsletter*, and through our website OASIS @ MAAP (www.aspergersyndrome.org). This organization keeps me in touch with thousands families in the United States and in 107 (so far) countries around the world. Those numbers increase weekly. As of this writing in April 2012, our website has had over 10 million visits and has only been live for two and a half years.

During the course of this work with families and teachers of more advanced individuals with autism spectrum disorders, I am often asked for brief, specific written information which explains in *plain language* what it means to be both "more advanced" and "disabled" (I prefer the new term "differently abled"). These requests prompted me to write my first version of this work (*High Functioning Individuals with Autism*). The change in accepted diagnostic terminology, the advancement of new information and therapies, and most importantly the fact that I have been more extensively educated by the many people who are challenged by autism spectrum disorders and who have communicated with me over these last few years, necessitated this newly updated version.

This book is an attempt to compile information gained from my parental experiences and through my studies on the subject, with the help of several excellent professional mentors, especially MAAP's Pro Advisory Board. More importantly, this book includes feedback received from parents and more advanced individuals who subscribe to my newsletter or whom I have met in my travels. This information can be used as a reference by those who deal regularly with more advanced individuals. All of the examples used in this book were relayed to me by these individuals or their parents, or are examples from my own life experiences.

Due to the diversity and complexity of the three DSM-IV-TR categories encompassed by my term "ASDs (autism spectrum disorders)," some of the characteristics or problems discussed may not be evident in the person you know. Use this book to find those characteristics and/or problems you *do* see, and then use relevant information and suggestions in whatever way is most beneficial. Also, be aware that the diagnostic criteria for all categories for pervasive developmental disorders will probably change in fewer than two years from now. Categories and "labels" may change, but the people about whom I am writing are *people* first. Let's just all figure out how to help them and leave the rest to the scientists (after hearing *plenty* of public feedback, of course).

For the sake of expediency, I shall alternate gender language when referring to individuals with ASDs. In addition, I shall simply say "the more advanced individual" or "the ASD individual," rather than saying "the more advanced individual with autism, Asperger syndrome, or pervasive developmental disorder—not otherwise specified." "More advanced" is not used in a pejorative manner—as if to say they are somehow better when referencing others on the autism spectrum—it simply refers to those with an autism spectrum challenge who can communicate in some form and are able to learn at a more age-appropriate rate if given proper supports. It is hoped that the information in this book will be helpful to all who are challenged with an ASD, not just those who are more able to show their abilities.

Chapter 1

What are Autism Spectrum Disorders?

Since the work in this book is based on the concept that more advanced individuals with autism, individuals with Asperger syndrome, and individuals with the label "pervasive developmental disorder—not otherwise specified" (PDD/NOS) are, in fact, all part of the autism spectrum, it is necessary to first define the syndrome of autism. Autism is a life-long developmental disability that typically is present at birth. It is called a developmental disability because it impairs the person's ability to develop at a normal rate in all areas of development and is most often diagnosed during the critical developmental years of early childhood, ages two to five years. Autism is referred to as a syndrome because it is a collection of symptoms, rather than a specific disease that can be identified by medical tests. There is no single, specific phenomenon that causes autism to occur. Instead, researchers suggest that there are various factors that lead to autism in different people.

Researchers do know that biochemical and structural brain abnormalities exist in many individuals with autism. These abnormalities may impair the brain's ability to process information, especially sensory information. The specific sensory mechanism affected may differ from individual to individual. In many, visual information may be processed typically, while auditory or tactile information may be processed atypically. In others, several or all forms of sensory information are inadequately or differently processed. The processing difficulties make the world a confusing place for these people. These abnormalities may also cause individuals with autism to experience movement disturbances. This may make their gait, posture, or other physical aspects appear awkward or otherwise different. Those interested in more information on movement disturbances in autism are encouraged to read materials by Dr. Anne Donnellan on this subject. Even if a more advanced individual does not appear to have a movement disturbance, Dr. Donnellan's materials make one think about an entirely different view of the subject of autism and differently abled people in general. However, some individuals with autism spectrum disorders (ASDs) are unusually agile and have good coordination skills in both gross and fine motor areas.

There are many behavioral symptoms that are accepted as indicating the presence of autism. However, identifying these symptoms in an individual *does not* always result in a reliable diagnosis. A reliable diagnosis of any of the ASDs should be determined by a team of professionals. See Chapter 3 for further information on diagnostic issues. The diagnosis of adults on the autism spectrum is even more complicated as many of their mannerisms and symptoms may have been successfully camouflaged over the years, as they have tried to fit in to non-spectrum society.

If possible, find professionals who have previous experience with individuals who have an ASD. It is quite difficult for a professional who doesn't see many cognitively average or above individuals with autism, Asperger syndrome, or PDD/NOS to diagnose them. With the ever-rising incidence rates for autism, terms such as "low incidence" should soon be erased from autism's vocabulary. Even those who have diagnosed and/or treated large numbers of more severely challenged individuals with autism often have difficulty in accurately diagnosing the more advanced individual, as that person's speech and ability to indicate a desire for or awareness of social interactions is so much more highly developed. When my daughter was diagnosed in 1975 she did not exhibit the rocking, flapping or other stereotypies that so many more severely challenged individuals with autism exhibit. However, those diagnosing her had seen several other children like her, so they knew that they were still dealing with someone within the autism spectrum.

Basically, the ASDs encompass the following traits:

1. onset of noticeable symptoms during early childhood

2. some type of difficulty in the production or use of verbal and/or non-verbal communication

3. evidence of rigidity in thought processes

4. difficulty with reciprocal social interaction.

Within those categories lie many variations of symptoms. However, the four areas are involved to some degree of different-than-typical ability in all individuals within the three DSM-IV-TR categories of autism, Asperger syndrome, and PDD/NOS. The proposed revisions in DSM-5 will combine social and communication skills into one category. The revisions may also call what I term as rigidity in thought processes to be "repetitive behaviors."

Two aspects of these conditions are important to remember. First, the conditions occur before or shortly after birth, although symptoms may not become evident until early childhood or even later in the case of extremely advanced individuals. Therefore, *autism spectrum challenges are not caused by poor parenting.* Second, *they are not curable, although they can be ameliorated in some individuals to the point of being no longer evident to the casual observer.* We all hope that some day medical research will give us more answers about cause that could lead to a cure, but so far the facts that are coming to light indicate that there may never be a cure. Symptoms can be greatly lessened, however. Although many have successfully adapted to meet the demands of their environment, I know of no properly documented cases in which an individual having one of the ASD diagnoses was completely cured. Therefore, parents and professionals must acknowledge that parents don't cause these disorders and that these are life-long conditions that will not disappear. I reiterate that "cure" and "highly adept" are very different things!

We must be careful in expressing our hopes for a cure because this hope is interpreted quite negatively by a lot of people with ASDs. They feel that their condition is an intrinsic aspect of their personalities—who they are. When they hear us talk of searching for a cure, they think we are trying to annihilate their personalities. I know I speak for all who care about people with ASDs challenges when I say that this is *not* our goal. We want to alleviate their suffering and make coping with everyday life easier for them.

Mary Anne Coppola, the mother of a young man diagnosed with autism, expressed this paradox quite well:

> Some days my greatest wish is that autism were to disappear from my son's life forever, and yet my son says that autism is who he is, and that is just fine with him. Erasing it would be like losing his arm or his eye. (Coppola, 1988)

As a parent of someone on the autism spectrum, I worry over the way genetic testing has led to some families seeking abortion and thus decreasing the rates of children born with Down syndrome. I know many wonderful people who have Down syndrome. I know their lives are difficult at times, but they are wonderful people to know and love. Do we want to create a world in which all people are the same?

Terms Within the "Spectrum"

The list of terms now used to identify individuals located at the higher end of the autism spectrum seems to be growing longer each day. Although it acknowledges the individuality of those being diagnosed, it serves to separate us out of a larger family we may need, as fellow travelers in a confusing land and as a political voice. Therefore, I feel that the term "autism" should be present. However, the following terms are either popular now or, in some cases, have been in the recent past. Therefore, reading materials on any of these subjects may be helpful and we will now enumerate them.

High-functioning autism, more able autism, near normal autism, mild autism, and socially aware autism are the terms that have, historically, encompassed the specific term "autism." Additional terms are Asperger syndrome (DSM-IV-TR), hyperlexia, non-verbal learning disorder, and PDD/NOS (DSM-IV-TR). A lot of this stemmed from the fact that until the past few years, most literature on autism (and *all* literature in the 1970s) concerns the more severely impaired individual. An irony is that Leo Kanner's original 11 case studies of people he termed "autistic" involved several individuals who were verbal and very communicative. After his writings, the majority of case studies were carried out in psychiatric institutions where only the more severe individuals were treated. This caused the literature and accepted standards for diagnosis to infer that most or all of those with autism were severely cognitively impaired and had very pronounced negative behaviors. Thus, parents who were trying to gain knowledge about their more advanced children felt these works did not accurately describe them. Professionals recognized this as well and new terms began to spring up.

It is important to note that Hans Asperger was writing his clinical description of individuals who seemed to share a common syndrome around the same time as Leo Kanner was writing his clinical description of individuals sharing a common set of challenges he was calling autism. In the DSM-IV-TR the central delineation used between autism and Asperger syndrome is sociability and articulate speech production. For more about the history of autism, read Adam Feinstein's book *A History of Autism* (2010).

The Asperger syndrome definition in DSM-IV-TR was greatly improved. Individuals with Asperger syndrome have more sociable behavior and more articulate speech, with seemingly little or no difficulty in language development. However, being able to produce articulate speech does not mean one can communicate well. The challenges in clear and effective communication experienced by *all* people on the autism spectrum result in difficulty with establishing and maintaining long-term friendships for people with Asperger syndrome, just as they do for other more advanced individuals.

From an outsider's view, the issue of "appropriateness" remains an issue in any of the ASD challenges. For example, an individual with one of these diagnoses may initially appear normal. After a period of time, he may engage in rude or some other form of socially inappropriate behavior, such as asking a stranger what type of underwear she is wearing, jumping into each unlocked car along a street and pretending to drive it, or asking a stranger how much money he makes.

This overlap of normal or above abilities with social impairment can create difficulties at every age and in many aspects of life. For example, as many lose some of the more extreme behavior symptoms associated with their challenge, professionals often misdiagnose them as having other disabilities or even mental illnesses. Since the average person will often see a more advanced individual behave in an apparently normal manner, they expect typical behavior at all times. When the individual exhibits unconventional behavior, it is misinterpreted as a deliberately odd or antisocial act. It is easy to see why many parents feel that their child's ability to achieve so much in spite of having an ASD challenge is both a blessing and a great difficulty.

Although individuals with any of the ASD diagnoses (autism, Asperger syndrome, autism disintegrative disorder, or PDD/NOS) exhibit the DSM-IV-TR criteria for their disability, some challenges may be more obvious than others.

To further complicate diagnostic issues, the proposed changes to the upcoming DSM-5 may eliminate the term "Asperger syndrome" as a diagnostic category and include it within autism. This is a highly controversial move that is eliciting highly emotional responses and firm rebuttals. Since this book will be completed before the final semantic issues are all finalized, I've chosen to address the currently used criteria. To view the proposed changes, go to www.dsm5.org. I am well acquainted with two professionals on the DSM-5 committee and can assure readers that they are people who care deeply about individuals with autism and firmly believe they are making diagnostic issues clearer, not more difficult.

We shall now look at the basic characteristics these diagnoses all *share*.

Onset of Symptoms

Symptoms that generally indicate that a child is not developing normally are not always evident in more advanced individuals during the first years of life. The more advanced individual may be able to use her intelligence to adapt responses to meet the demands of the environment. In some instances, subtle symptoms are not apparent until more sophisticated social skills are called for in a preschool or kindergarten setting. Regardless, many parents report that symptoms were not evident until their child reached three or four years of age. In the case of extremely advanced individuals, symptoms may not be recognized until the late teen or adult years. In some cases, the newborn infant was "too good," seemingly content to be all alone, in some cases to the point of not even crying when hungry or wet. In other cases, the infant was frequently distraught with bouts of "keening" or other signs of inconsolable distress. These crying or keening incidents seem to start without an antecedent and can last many hours, with all conventional efforts to comfort them failing miserably.

Impairment in Communication Skills

The majority of more advanced ASD individuals can articulate speech clearly. However, a small percentage (notably those who are severely hearing impaired) use little or no speech. When first learning to speak, many individuals (especially those with a diagnosis of autism) use echolalia (see Glossary). Echolalia is the act of repeating verbatim what one has heard said. Though not all echolalia is communicative, many repeat whole sentences word for word with some intention of communication. Those who have echolalia usually lose it through maturity and good language/communication therapy, or it becomes so sophisticated that it is difficult to detect. Echolalia may reappear, especially when the individual is under stress.

Most people with ASDs who are highly intelligent have and use a large and articulate vocabulary, but do not always know where and how to use it, and with whom. For example, when my daughter was in second grade, she knew the meaning and correct spelling of words like "apogee" and "gibbous," but she couldn't express many simple needs and feelings.

Individuals with ASDs may "talk at" people about their obsessive interests for prolonged periods of time, with absolutely no awareness that the listener is totally uninterested in what is being said. In most of these instances, giving them subtle social cues, such as repeatedly looking at the clock and sighing, is futile.

Even the most articulate person with an ASD may encounter problems when engaging in a conversation, such as volume control, turn-taking, appropriate verbal responses in conversations, and knowing when to begin and end a conversation. Their interpretation of the written, spoken, and non-verbal communication of others is often very different from non-autism-spectrum interpretation. Some use and interpret communication in a very literal and rigid manner, making it difficult for them to interpret words or stories with double meanings, and to identify and endure teasing. However, others with ASD challenges use humor (look up Canadian Jason McElwain's comedy), teasing, and double meaning in jokes and other aspects of life. Many love to use puns.

A parent in California wrote that her son (who is diagnosed as a more advanced person with autism) gave her a graphic example of his literalness. When exhorting him to remember to do something as others would do it, she often said, "You want to act normal, don't you?" At this point, her son always assured her that he did indeed want to "act normal." Then one day, after a particularly frustrating incident, she said, "Do you know what 'normal' really means?" "Yes," he replied, "it is the second button from the left on the washing machine." We might ask ourselves whether or not the young man was impaired in his ability to interpret her communication or whether she was unwise in the words she chose to use with a person who has ASD (Richards, 1992).

Many of the communication challenges facing the more advanced individual are illustrated by this quote from a young man who has ASD:

> When I was in high school I would hear other people say things which were accepted well. Then I would make the same type of remark, but often there was an exchange of glances. People might say, "Get out of here." Or somebody would take my remarks and try to fit them in.
>
> Now when I interact in a group and am accepted in a normal way, I feel as though it is some kind of rare victory. Usually I try not to say anything unless I am asked a direct question. Even then I sometimes get glances because I say far too much. I don't know when to stop, when I have said enough to answer the question well. (Dewey and Everard, 1974)

The same young man replies to the interviewer's suggestion that he try to improve his *listening* skills and to use the words and phrases of those with whom he is speaking as a guide to answering their questions.

> Now I have good hearing and I think I listen well. But sometimes I latch on to the wrong words as most important and shut out the ones the other person thought were important. It is not a question of hearing the words, but of knowing what is important in the situation and what the other person assumes I already know. (Dewey and Everard, 1974)

This young man's comment about "what the other person assumes I already know" addresses the skills many professionals identify as "shared knowledge" and "perspective taking." I refer to these two skills as "social repertoire." People typically gain social repertoire through observing and experiencing life. The observed social repertoire utilized during specific events is internalized and reserved for future use. This learned social repertoire guides us when we communicate with others and when we interpret the communications we receive from others. These many and various "facts of life" are invaluable in understanding the gist of conversation and social interaction in general.

People with ASDs often have difficulty generalizing information, in particular *social* information. In other words, "learning a lesson" (or at least what a "non-spectrum person" (see Glossary) would judge as an appropriate lesson) from a specific social experience and then applying the information to a different situation in an appropriate manner may be problematic. Therefore, many cognitively advanced individuals with ASDs have a more limited amount and/or less appropriate (according to the judgment of non-spectrum people) use of generalized information in their repertoires. This makes speaking and understanding what is said in social interactions even more difficult.

In addition to the conversational aspects of their communications, these individuals often speak with an unusual cadence, a stilted manner, an odd timbre, and/or poor volume control (either too softly or too loudly, varying from instance to instance). When a person with an ASD speaks, it often sounds as though she has rehearsed what she is saying. In fact, it is through rehearsal that many people with ASDs learn appropriate things to say in a variety of different settings.

Many cognitively advanced people have problems answering questions (either verbally or in writing) that require abstract or conceptual answers, such as essay questions in school. At times they appear to get stuck mid-sentence, or may repeat the part where they got stuck several times before stopping or moving on. My daughter often hesitates for long periods of time mid-sentence when telling a story. This sometimes leads us to believe she is finished, when in fact she is stuck. Others will then continue conversing with or around her, causing her to feel insulted and ignored.

Often the more upset ASD individuals feel, the less able they are to tell anyone what is upsetting them. Since communication may be more difficult when most needed, these individuals often end up angry and frustrated. Temper tantrums, inappropriate or irrelevant speech, aggression, or other forms of behavior deemed inappropriate by non-spectrum people may result from this anger and frustration.

Repetitive verbal arguments and/or repetitive verbal questions can occur during angry, confusing, or frustrating times. The agitated ASD individual may make a statement or ask a question in an argumentative fashion over and over again for prolonged periods of time. It can feel as though the person with autism is actually engaging in a more sophisticated temper tantrum. Attempts to logically and rationally answer their questions and arguments usually fail. Suggestions for dealing with these repetitive verbal behaviors can be found in Chapter 6. Another aspect of communication that presents major difficulties for the more advanced individual is non-verbal communication.

Typically, people communicate with more than just their words. They communicate through gestures, facial expressions, vocal prosody (see Glossary), sighs or other noises, body stance, and proximity to the person addressed. For example, if the content of someone's conversation is irritating, you may sigh, squirm in your chair, or stare up into the sky as if asking a greater power for assistance. More advanced individuals often have trouble using and interpreting these forms of non-verbal communication. As one young man reported, "People send each other messages with their eyes and I don't understand those messages" (Newson, 1980).

Ironically, despite many challenges with communication, a significant number of more advanced individuals have exceptional skills in the area of learning and using foreign languages. One young man from Switzerland, who speaks German, French, and English, and who is very talented in playing the piano said, "I think of language as music...the music of the nations...the music of mankind" (Fischer, 1997). I've no idea how this man speaks in person, since I've not had the privilege of meeting him in person, but he certainly has profound thoughts! It is important to remember that challenges in communication do *not* mean that an individual isn't sensitive and intelligent and doesn't have a lot of worthwhile thoughts to share with others.

Non-spectrum readers should now take time to reflect on these communication differences and use them to change future communications with more advanced individuals and to better understand future communications from them. As non-spectrum people we certainly ascribe to the theory that communication is a two-way street!

Qualitative Impairment in Reciprocal Social Interaction

Social cognition (see Glossary) and social skills differences are regarded by many professionals as the true core challenge of ASDs. Individuals who have received a diagnosis of Asperger syndrome or PDD/NOS usually *appear* more socially fluid and curious than those who have been recently diagnosed as more advanced individuals with autism. The former individuals more frequently initiate a seemingly more fluid social contact, but often have an awkwardness or inappropriateness about this interaction. Although more advanced individuals with autism may appear withdrawn, aloof, and/or uninterested in their peers or people in general, many of them need and want friends very much. The definitive difference diagnostically between autism and Asperger syndrome has been normal language development or language delay. Characteristics such as poor eye contact, ineffective or inappropriate body language, tactile defensiveness, difficulty with empathy, and poor conversational skills contribute to the aloof appearance of cognitively advanced individuals with either diagnosis. It seems as though general improvement in communication and behavior sets the stage for an increased desire to be with and interact with other people. It may be that improved communication skills and less distracting behavior simply make it easier for the more advanced person with autism to convey this need for friends. However, too often they find themselves observers or victims of society, rather than easy participants in the same.

No two individuals of *any* commonality are exactly alike. The same is true of these unique people. Many are very socially precocious. Others appear aloof and uninterested in social interaction. Some want to socialize, but don't know how to be successful at it. Others simply do not want to interact with others. This can be because they are uncomfortable trying to interact or because of past frustration, pain, and/or failure in social efforts.

Unfortunately, the increased interest in making friends that frequently occurs during the adolescent years does not coincide with an increased ability to make and maintain friendships. Occasionally, the more advanced individual will respond positively to friendly approaches from peers and may even initiate or participate in forming a friendship. However, their lack of experience and skill in *maintaining* friendships too often brings these tentative relationships to an end. This brings additional pain and sorrow to the adolescent and his family.

There are many things the family can do for their child who has ASD, but creating and maintaining friendships for them is exceptionally challenging. Typically, only a few rare and special individuals maintain close friendships with individuals who have ASDs for prolonged periods of time.

People who have tried and failed in their attempts at making and maintaining a friendship with a person with an ASD often feel they gave a lot and received very little in return. What most don't realize is that they have, in fact, received a lot from the challenged person—but the behavior and actions they see don't reflect the enormous effort the more advanced person had to expend to respond to the friendship appropriately. Also, the friend of the challenged person gains *as a person* in ways they may not, at first, realize. My daughter's friends feel as though they have gained more sensitivity towards others, a greater ability to clearly communicate and a greater appreciation for many of the smaller aspects of their life, such as personal freedom and innate empathy, which they possess without effort and the individual with an ASD struggles to attain.

My daughter was included (see Glossary) in a typical school and typical classrooms within the public school system since second grade. I have noted that many of her peers who originally befriended her were somewhat more intelligent than most. My theory is not that kindness and intelligence are somehow correlated. I think that people who are very gifted and talented know what it feels like to be different. This may mean they feel more empathy towards others whom they perceive as also different.

A few of these peers have continued to be friends with my daughter, but these friendships have changed through the years. Many have become what I would describe as "tolerantly friendly," but none continue to regard her as a "best friend" or continue to contact her on a regular basis, with the exception of three women who knew her in high school. One knew her through the music program and as a scholastic tutor who became her roommate after they had both graduated from college. My daughter was living in a large apartment in the community where this young woman wanted to work. She lived with my daughter for one year, until her marriage. She was a friendly, cheerful roommate and friend, although she spent very limited time with my daughter while there. I think that part of this was due to her very busy schedule and the other part was (perhaps) that she needed other friends who were more able to be innately empathic with her.

In college, my daughter made many new and supportive friends. They demonstrated exceptional tolerance and acceptance of those qualities that make her different. They tended to include her more in their social gatherings and accept her outbursts and other "incidents" more easily than her peers in high school. Perhaps this was due to the information they received prior to her arrival on campus concerning her disability and her need for friends. Perhaps it was the increased maturity of those peers. Her relationship with an exceptionally popular student who was her friend and math tutor in high school also helped her from the very beginning of her freshman year in college. This wonderful young woman took her to any and all of her social outings during the first few months of college. This relationship signaled to others that it was socially acceptable to befriend my daughter. In fact, if this young woman asked if our daughter could come with her to a party and was told no, she didn't attend the party. Since she was very popular—people wanted her there and were more prone to including my daughter. This young woman is now middle-aged and has her own family, but still regards my daughter as one of her closest friends. She and her family have become a part of our family. She continues to love our daughter as a "sister."

The last continuing friend that I'll mention actually knew our daughter in grade school and befriended her then. She continued that friendship through high school. They were separated in college, due to different schools and activities. This girl didn't come home for summer vacations. They were reunited as adults and have resumed the friendship, to the delight of both parties.

The qualities in my daughter most frequently cited by her peers as making her worthy of friendship include intelligence, loyalty, and her areas of exceptional ability and interest. I also suspect that peers sense her innocence and vulnerability and seek to protect her.

Despite successful experiences, each year people slip away from this friendly peer group. Although others eventually replace those she has lost, to my daughter it seems as though every peer she learns to care about and trust leaves her just when she begins to become secure in the friendship. This attrition is sometimes due to misunderstood events and/or characteristics that are part of my daughter's autism, but are instead perceived as the actions of a spoiled, overprotected brat who is deliberately self-centered. In other cases, people move, marry, and/or have children, which changes their social circle and interests.

For example, difficulty in sorting and processing sensory information makes situations involving a lot of noise and movement disconcerting to many individuals with autism. When my daughter was in high school, I was talking to a group of her peers and explaining that she wanted and needed friendship and encouragement from each of them. One of the peers commented, "You tell us that she wants our friendship, but when we say 'Hi' to her in the halls, she doesn't even look up or answer us. I don't call that very friendly. I think *you* just want her to have friends." I quickly explained that my daughter wasn't replying to this girl or her friends in the halls because of the noise and fast movement around her, making the halls a very difficult and even frightening place. My daughter probably didn't see or hear these people because she was focused on navigating the hall without losing her composure. This explanation was accepted with a little skepticism, and then a lot of relief, by the peer. But what about all the others in the school who didn't hear the explanation and thought my daughter was an unconcerned snob? It is easy to see how more advanced individuals become the target for rejection and cruelty from their peers due to similar misunderstandings.

Most people with ASDs have trouble tolerating last-minute changes in plans. Social plans are frequently made by non-spectrum people at the last moment. People with ASDs need a few days to process and adapt to changes in their routine. Therefore, when someone calls them in the morning and asks them to do something that they may really like that evening, they will usually say no and be somewhat distressed that they were even asked. If they receive a social invitation with (preferably) a week's notice, then they have several days to work out how they will adapt to the change in their routine. Conversely, they may fail to give reasonable notice when they want to make social plans for themselves with others. For instance, my daughter decided to have a St. Patrick's Day party to commemorate her first St. Pat's in her new apartment. She elaborately made food and beverage plans for several weeks in advance, but did not invite anyone until a day or two before. Since the people she asked had all made other plans by then, she had only one guest, who had to sit with her as she grieved the failure of her much-anticipated party. As her parent, I try to learn of such plans and prompt her to proper action at the proper time. Sometimes, I even call a few of her friends myself. However, I realize that I won't always be there to do this for her, so I must help her adapt by making some generalized rules about how to have a successful party. For my daughter and *most* cognitively advanced

ASD people, these rules must be written down. It is often a good way to properly process and use the rules.

The area of making friends is particularly critical to learning social skills for the more advanced individual. When peers continue to interact with him in a positive manner, they can model and teach age-appropriate interactions, dress, and interests that cannot be taught by someone not in that age group.

The difficulties that more advanced individuals experience in relating to others were described by one mother:

> We are fortunate that our son has always attended a regular school. He has even taken gifted math and science classes the past two years in junior high. Yet, this bright boy cannot verbally relate a simple personal experience or engage in a friendly conversation. In his preschool and elementary years, he was quite content to be alone, to draw endless maps and mazes, happy in his private bubble. However, recently some gradual changes have been occurring. After so many years, he now wants friends, and seems to be experiencing loneliness for the first time in his life. Yet using the phone to call a friend is a sometimes insurmountable task. After years of not even recognizing that another human being was in the same room, he is now beginning to look outward to people for the first time and not knowing how to reach them brings frustration and sadness not only to him, but to me.
>
> He hasn't the vaguest idea how to initiate a new friendship. He can only watch from afar and hope that someone approaches him. This is very painful in the junior high years when social relationships are so critical, and his behavior is so often misunderstood.
>
> How do you teach a 14-year-old those basic social graces we think of as second nature? He often does not respond when even someone he knows well says "Hi!" He has trouble choosing from a restaurant menu and requesting his selection from the waitress. "Please" and

"Thank you" are usually forgotten. He rarely asks questions or even appears to be curious about people. Yet he wants to be with others and included in their activities. Their rejection has caused him to withdraw into isolation again. Trying to be "normal" has been so painful. As thrilled as I am to see that he is finally reaching out, I remember the happy, carefree boy who lived in a private world, and I cry to watch the sad, vulnerable teenager who has taken his place. (Coppola, 1988)

Even when an ASD individual receives years of excellent help and strives to reach his potential, the area of social skills and social knowledge remain difficult. Included in the concept of reciprocal social interaction is social empathy—the ability to take the perspective of another person. Fortunately, a deep understanding of another person's views and feelings is not necessarily identified by society as "normal" behavior. A general comprehension of and reaction to another's perspective is sufficient. When the more advanced individual attempts to do this, he often fails. Many more advanced people appear to have either great difficulty with or an inability to identify accurately the emotions expressed by the facial expressions and body language of others.

Perhaps this lack of success in reading the perspectives and emotions of others leads the more advanced individual to stop trying to see things from another's perspective. Whatever the cause, awareness of the perspective of others is a challenge for most people with ASDs.

As noted earlier, ASD individuals may be more able to express social relatedness through written communication. For example, one young man wrote an interesting rebuttal to the concept that people with ASDs lack social empathy. In his letter, he aptly interconnects social empathy and communication:

I keep reading that people on the spectrum lack empathy and are unable to take others' perspectives. I think it might be more fair to say that they lack certain expressive and receptive communication skills, possibly including some basic instincts that make communication a natural process for most people, and that this, combined with any cognitive or perceptual differences, means that people with ASD do not share others' perceptions. "Empathy" is a nebulous term that is often used to mean projection of one's own feelings onto others; it is therefore much easier to "empathize" with (i.e. to understand the feelings of) someone whose perceptions are very different. But if empathy means being able to understand a perspective that is different from one's own, then it is not possible to determine how much empathy is present without first having an adequate understanding of each person's perspective and of how different those perspectives are from each other.

... But I do mind when in spite of so much effort, I still miss cues, and someone who has much better inherent communication ability than I do but who has not even taken a close enough look at my perspective to notice the enormity of the chasm between us tells me that my failure to understand is because I lack "empathy." If I know that I do not understand people and I devote all this energy and effort to figuring them out, do I have more or less empathy than people who not only do not understand me, but who do not even notice that they don't understand me? (Sinclair, 1989)

Markedly Restricted Repertoire of Activities and Interests (Evidence of Rigidity in Thought Processes)

I prefer to discuss the "restricted repertoire" aspect of ASDs under what I feel is a more accurate and encompassing concept—evidence of rigidity in thought processes. A number of easily misunderstood behaviors provide us with evidence that ASD individuals experience rigidity of thought processes. These behaviors include:

- repetitive verbal arguments
- resistance to change
- ritualistic behavior
- obsessive interests.

Repetitive verbal arguments and/or repetitive verbal questions are exhibited by many ASD individuals. As mentioned earlier, this behavior may indicate frustration, fear, confusion, desire to maintain social interaction, the existence of echolalia, or a feeling of loss of control in certain situations. This behavior can be extremely aggravating to others. During a repetitive verbal argument or question, these individuals may resort to a recurring theme in arguing with or questioning those around them. It should be stressed that this behavior is typically a means of communicating frustration or distress and is rarely valid and often only loosely related to what is actually disrupting the individual. Therefore, repeatedly and logically answering the questions or the logic of the argument will not always help.

The more advanced individual is usually resistant to change. New environments and changes in routine may upset him. However, some begin to enjoy travel as they grow older and derive great joy in planning trips, even if only day-long events. In many instances, their enjoyment results from planning the details of the trip (e.g., reading the maps, learning about the climate statistics of the area, memorizing facts about the area), rather than the execution of travel plans.

A smaller percentage of individuals manifest ritualistic behavior, such as demanding the same foods for breakfast every day, demanding that the same conversation take place before bed every night, or needing to dress in the same order of succession of clothing each day (e.g., socks first, then undershirt, etc.). To a lesser degree, ritualistic behavior may be reflected in an insistence on routine. Often this routine is perceived only by them. If the people involved in such a routine fail to notice it as such, difficulties may follow. For example, when my daughter started college, she left on a Thursday. By the next Wednesday, I felt I should stop in to check on her adjustment—both mental and physical—to school. I followed through with a visit. I established that I would visit once a week to help her with laundry and to attend to any problems she might be having. The next week, Wednesday turned out to be the best day for me to visit, so I again went down on that day. After that, if I did not visit on a Wednesday, she was very agitated until she saw me. It didn't matter how many times she was reminded that I *would* be down to see her that week, she felt she *must* see me on Wednesdays.

Many ASD individuals have some area of interest in which they are highly informed, obsessively interested, and/or exceptionally talented. In many cases if good teaching and mentoring are used, these talents and interests can eventually be expanded and somewhat redirected into employable skills or at least life-long hobbies.

However, some individuals have one exceptional area of skill, but lack a majority of other tangential skills that make the skill employable, as well as the skills of daily semi-independent living. Many years ago, professionals referred to these isolated types of skills as "islands of knowledge" or "islands of precocity." Despite efforts to make our society more sensitive to insulting or downgrading terms in reference to challenged individuals, sometimes these individuals are still today referred to as "autistic (or idiot) savants." These terms refer to the disparity between highly developed skills in some areas and low skill development in other areas. Basically, this is an archaic and insulting term to most individuals on the autism spectrum.

Although the individual may lack many social and/or self-help skills, he may excel in areas such as music or math. A person with an ASD may have no measurable standard mathematical abilities, but be a "calendar manipulator." Calendar manipulators can, for example, reliably state the exact date for the third Tuesday in March in the year 2058 within seconds of being asked that question for the first time. Others can multiply four-digit numbers in their heads in seconds, but may not be able to calculate accurately the change at a cash register. Some display incredible musical talents. One young man can perform long, intricate piano music pieces played for him only once. The areas of exceptional ability vary from person to person. Curiously, as they gain in social and self-help skills, many ASD individuals lose some degree of their exceptional skills or lose an exceptional skill altogether.

Other Areas of Consideration and Relevance

Although disruptive or inappropriate behaviors are an aspect of ASDs, they are not behavior disorders. The occurrence of inappropriate behavior is perhaps the most heartbreaking problem for family members of the person with an ASD. For example, these individuals may make odd noises or laugh unusually at unpredictable intervals despite gains in other areas. At times they may grimace oddly or stare off into space while appearing totally unaware of what is going on around them. This can lead people to conclude that they are eccentric or choosing to be strange.

We often refer to individuals who suffer from one of the ASDs as having an "invisible disability." When provided with sufficient training, these individuals are capable of acting "normal" for prolonged periods of time. In addition, they have no physical anomalies associated with their disability. In fact, they are quite often exceptionally attractive people. Often, without warning, unusual behaviors occur. These outbursts or inappropriate behaviors become a greater problem as the person ages and matures. After overcoming the many obstacles caused by this condition, ASD individuals are more able to express a desire to be with people other than immediate family members. Therefore, they tend to be "out" in typical society more frequently. Suddenly a behavior change occurs that causes shock, disbelief, and misjudgment by those who either do not know the individual well or do not understand the characteristics of an ASD individual. Those registering negative reactions to this inappropriate behavior can range from special education teachers to friends, extended family members, and community members.

In summary, ASD individuals are often shunned and criticized for behaviors that are an inherent condition of autism, Asperger syndrome, or PDD/NOS, simply because those around them do not understand that the behaviors are part of the disability. For example, if a blind person stumbles and breaks a piece of furniture, those who witness it know that this incident was a result of the individual's blindness. Their reaction would most likely be compassion. Conversely, if an ASD person has to wait for a late bus, she may become very upset and act inappropriately. Observers may believe the person is just being deliberately rude.

This confusion and these negative reactions create frustration and further heartbreak for the ASD individual, his parents, and siblings. The mother of an ASD person put this quandary into words (please note that this quote was given in 1982 when language like "abnormal" was used for lack of better and more sensitive descriptors):

> I think I'd rather have had a *normal* abnormal child, if you know what I mean. If one has [a child with a visible handicap]…you know the child's only going to go so far, and that's that. And the child's obviously not normal, and people say "Ah, what a shame, what a pity…" but with an [ASD] child, you never know from one day to the next, nobody *recognizes* them as abnormal, and you just don't know what to do; and really there are no rules, so you just do the best you can. (Newson, Dawson and Everard, 1982)

Contrary to popular myth, some ASD individuals can become verbally and/or physically aggressive. This is important to note since school psychologists and others have disputed using the autism spectrum labels for the ASD individual who demonstrates the characteristics of autism, Asperger syndrome, or PDD/NOS when aggression is present. In these individuals, aggression is most likely to surface during puberty. They may be labeled as having oppositional defiant disorder, or as being bipolar.

Many ASD individuals show patterns of regression and/or depression during adolescence. In some cases the depression can lead to suicide attempts. The regression can last from a few months to several years. When this difficult time is over, behavior often mellows considerably and the person may greatly increase his ability to learn and grow, both scholastically and socially. Sadly, this increase in learning ability often takes place after the opportunity for free access to public schooling has past. As the ASD child matures, traditional behavior management methods may become ineffective. Parents and "hands-on" professionals will need to adopt subtler and/or more sophisticated methods of behavior support. These behavioral strategies should be positive and should take into account the difficulty any person has in changing basic behavior patterns. Positive programming focuses on teaching appropriate behaviors to replace inappropriate or problem behaviors (Donnellan *et al.*, 1988). Parents become participants in identifying desirable alternative behaviors that fit the demands of each individual's home, school, and community environments.

The loss, lessening, or modification of "classic" behaviors associated with autism (e.g., echolalia, lack of eye contact, stereotypic movements, or temper tantrums) can lead professionals trying to make a diagnosis to an inappropriate conclusion. Professionals are trained to base their diagnoses on observable behaviors, not on parental recollections of past behaviors associated with ASDs. They may incorrectly decide that the person cannot have an ASD challenge.

A rapid increase in accomplishments and a decrease in abrasive behavior problems can lead professionals to conclude that the person is "cured." In other cases, a claim is made that the individual has "grown out of their autism." These false claims often cause great disappointment for the family when the individual manifests new problems related to his disability. These claims of cures may be heard by other parents of ASD individuals and false hopes may be generated about an approach that may "cure" their loved one. Parents of ASD individuals need information, understanding, and encouragement, not false hope! Dr. Temple Grandin is a famous woman who has autism. I've been privileged to know Temple since she was in graduate school (mostly via phone, but later in person). Many people regard Temple as cured. Temple is brilliant and extremely accomplished. She has authored multiple books on autism issues and is a highly regarded engineer in the field of animal science. Yet, to refer to her highly evolved skills and restraint as a cure, belies her struggles to maintain decorum and the level of behavior expected from her now at all times.

Every time my daughter masters a new skill or overcomes an ASD mannerism or behavior, I find myself wanting to believe that she will make it all the way—that maybe someday she will be regarded by that most wonderful and frustrating of all terms, "normal." But then I plant my feet firmly on the ground and realize that autism, Asperger syndrome, and PDD/NOS as we know them now, are not—and may never be—curable conditions. I am both comforted and challenged by the fact that there seem to be endless possibilities to what my daughter *can* accomplish. I am grateful for her potential and for what she has already overcome. In the midst of optimism, I constantly worry about her future and the unknown challenges she must face.

Chapter 2

Terms Frequently used to Describe Individuals on the Autism Spectrum

ASD Individual

ASD is an abbreviation of "autism spectrum disorder." This term refers to individuals with all of the more advanced spectrum of autism conditions. It encompasses autism, Asperger syndrome, and pervasive developmental disorder—not otherwise specified. It is merely a more concise way of referring to this group. In this book, I use the term in reference to more advanced individuals within the autism spectrum.

Asperger Syndrome

In the mid-1980s, I took an informal survey about which term parents preferred. Approximately half of the parents who responded preferred this term to the others. In most cases, this was because it does not have the word "autism" in it. These parents felt that the term "autism" suggests that people with this disorder are withdrawn, non-verbal, and self-abusive. This adamant belief led to the inclusion of the term in DSM-IV-TR.

High-functioning People with Autism

This term indicates the dichotomy of these individuals. On the one hand, they have great difficulties; on the other, they have the serious challenge of autism. It was, until recently, the term of choice for most professionals.

Hyperlexia

Most neuropsychology texts use this term simply to refer to an accelerated *ability* to read. However, some groups use it as a name for a disability when the mechanical reading ability exceeds the ability to comprehend. I feel this term further fragments families of more advanced ASD individuals into yet another political group. However, the American Hyperlexia Association uses this term and has truly excellent teaching programs.

More Able Person with Autism

I formerly used this term in my newsletter. I felt it reflected the comparable potential of these individuals. However, I feel that this term reflects negatively on those with autism who do not *appear* to be as able, as though saying they lack potential. For many, this potential is only recently being explored. All individuals with autism have ability. It is difficult to rate ability.

More Advanced Individual

This term isn't as judgmental as More Able Person with Autism, therefore I find it preferable.

Non-verbal Learning Disorder

This term refers to the learning challenges faced by individuals with Asperger syndrome. It refers to generally impaired social and environmental learning challenges.

Pervasive Developmental Disorder— Not Otherwise Specified

Talk about vague terminology—I suggest it would be better to use the term "I'm not sure folks!" This term usually refers to a very highly skilled person (compared with autism or even Asperger syndrome) who has very good language, vocabulary, and articulation and who also shows a lot of social precocity. However, these individuals still have problems with appropriate social reciprocity. Technically, it means someone with some, but not all, of the essential symptoms of autism.

The previous sections have presented a simplified description of a very complex condition. The following chapter focuses on what you can *do* to help an ASD person in their home, school, and community environments.

Chapter 3

The Younger ASD
Individual at Home

Recognizing and Diagnosing the Problem

The first time that parents need help with or become concerned about their child is when that child's behavior becomes odd or problematic. This may occur soon after birth or it may not occur until the child is several years old. The first indicators of an ASD will vary according to the individual child and his parents. Some of these children are very placid as babies. They cry little or not at all. Many do not indicate even extreme hunger. Others are prone to frequent episodes of seemingly inconsolable crying. When parents try to comfort the crying infant through holding and rocking, they may find the child responds by pushing away or becoming rigid. Parents of this latter group usually are aware of a problem at an earlier age. Pediatricians may decide that the child has colic or that the parents are just being over-anxious about their child. If they receive medicine to reduce the effects of colic, it often is either totally ineffective or has the opposite reaction of making the infant even more irritable. Initially, parents of placid babies think they have a very "good baby." Later, they notice that with this placidity comes a marked indifference to parents and siblings. Usually, these children do not go through the normal developmental stage of being afraid of strangers or they go through this stage in a prolonged and severe form. Most don't reach to be picked up as babies. They also don't point to objects that they want, but may take a parent's hand or arm and reach it toward the desired object. In other children, there may be no noticeable differences until they reach preschool or kindergarten, when they must interact with other children in a group setting.

Cues to the problems of ASDs can be very obvious in some cases and in others so subtle that the parents (no matter how experienced in child rearing or how caring and concerned they are) do not acknowledge these behaviors as cues to a more serious problem. Therefore, some parents seek a diagnosis or assistance for their child at a very early age and others do not seek professional help until the child is three years or older. In an increasing number of cases, people or their family members discover their ASD as adults in middle age or beyond.

"Don't worry so much," "Just relax and learn to enjoy your child," "Don't expect so much from your child," "What you really need is a brother or sister for little_____," "You need to use better discipline on you child." These are typical comments that parents of more advanced children hear from friends, family, and trusted professionals, especially their family pediatrician. These pieces of advice are not only useless, they are also frustrating and destructive to caring parents who are genuinely concerned about a very real problem (see Appendix A).

In our case, my husband and I felt there was something wrong with our daughter from the third day of her life. We felt she had an unusual cry and did not easily relate to us. Since we were new parents, physicians and family told us that our inexperience as parents made us *think* there was a problem and that the only problem was our ineptitude.

The parents of more cognitively advanced ASD children or adults frequently experience multiple misdiagnoses, or never receive an accurate diagnosis until many years after their search begins. Accurately diagnosing autism spectrum challenges must be done via multidisciplinary, clinical assessment. Parents who are fortunate enough to receive an accurate diagnosis for their child during early childhood are somewhat ahead of the game. Remember, a diagnosis does not always delineate programming or service needs, but it can provide direction. It is hoped that by reading this book, one may get enough descriptive information to decide whether or not to seek a full diagnosis, if necessary.

Once a diagnosis of autism, Asperger syndrome, or pervasive developmental disorder—not otherwise specified is made, parents begin to determine what they can do to help their child. The following recommendations are based on personal experience and the experiences of other parents with whom I have interacted.

Recommendations for Families with Children or Teens

Further Workups

When parents or professionals suspect a child may have one of the ASDs, they should seek a thorough evaluation performed by a team of professionals. This team may include a pediatrician (preferably a developmental pediatrician), a pediatric neurologist, a psychiatrist or psychologist who is well versed in the full ASD spectrum, a communication specialist, and an occupational therapist. Hospital or university affiliated clinics often offer these services. Costs vary greatly, but many operate on a sliding-fee scale. Evaluation by a multidisciplinary team is advisable because suggestions that represent different perspectives can best begin to address the diverse programming needs of the child.

Services that are available to the preschool-age child, either through itinerant services in the home or through direct services in a school or other facility, may be recommended. Therapists and teachers can teach parents games and exercises that can be performed with their child in the home. These are often fun and provide parents with the rewarding experience of feeling they are finally helping their child. Any parent of a child with autism will tell you that it is very frustrating to want to do something—anything—to help one's child, yet to receive no specific direction by professionals as to what that something might be.

POSITIVE BEHAVIOR SUPPORTS

A common recommendation given by diagnostic facilities is that parents learn and use behavior management approaches, which are currently referenced as positive behavior supports. To ensure continuity, these techniques should be used both at home and in school. Using such principles can be an enormous help in restoring some order to your family life in addition to helping a child's behavior improve. The most important aspect of this approach is that it must be used in a reasonably consistent manner and it should be *positive*. By this, I mean it should focus more on teaching appropriate behavior than on decreasing inappropriate behavior.

When beginning to use positive behavioral supports, some caution must be exerted. Parents of children challenged by ASD were born no stronger, braver, or nobler than anyone else— despite what some people would like to believe and make parents believe! When using behavior management strategies at home, parents should decide what they can and will expect of themselves. Although parents should try to be as consistent as possible, there will be days when they are simply too tired to be consistent, for example, the time to follow through coincides with a fire in the dryer; or one of the other children swallows a goldfish. The authors of positive behavior support books usually fail to realize that despite your full, sincere efforts to help your ASD child, you still are expected by your other children and spouse to fulfill the traditional roles of housekeeper, nurse, home repairer, cook, breadwinner, etc.

To sum up, learn about positive behavior supports to whatever extent you are able, but don't berate yourself if your experiences don't go by the book. Be aware that current research and practices in behavioral therapy emphasize that positive techniques are the ones that have the most lasting effects. *Don't use punishment* as a behavior management technique. You may be modeling a behavior (punishment) that your child will use one day—on you! Focus on teaching an appropriate behavior, rather than merely eliminating a problem behavior.

There are many books available on this subject. However, they are often long and highly technical. Two excellent and short books about behavior management are *Asperger Syndrome and Difficult Moments* (Myles and Southwick, 2005) and *Progress Without Punishment* (Donnellan *et al.*, 1988).

OTHER THERAPIES

The number of therapies available for people with ASDs now numbers in the dozens. A good discussion of many of these therapies can be found in:

- *The Oasis Guide to Asperger Syndrome* (Bashe and Kirby, 2001)
- *The Parents' Guide to Teaching Kids with Asperger Syndrome and Similar ASDs* (Bashe, 2011)
- *Pervasive Developmental Disorders* (Waltz, 1999).

In selecting other possible therapies for your child, you should consider the unique characteristics (both strengths and challenges) of your child, your financial ability to afford the therapy, whether your school can carry out this therapy within the context of the school day, and any possible negative aspects of the therapy. Beware of any therapy that suggests it is *the only* answer for all children with any form of ASD! Certainly beware of any therapy or program that promises a cure or mentions others who have been cured by its approach. This simply is not true and suggests these therapies may manipulate the families whom they serve. Look for therapies and programs that are honest and open about their approaches and any possible problems.

Respite

Helping an ASD loved one develop into the best and happiest person she can be is an experience filled with rewards and *many* challenges. The accomplishments achieved by the child bring great joy. The challenges bring tremendous fatigue and stress. These problems will not defeat the parent or child if the parent remains realistic about their own needs as an individual. A parent is more than just a mom or dad. She is a unique personality. If a parent doesn't take care of herself, both physically and emotionally, how well will she take care of her child?

I am not suggesting that, on hearing the child's diagnosis, parents run off to some tropical beach for a relaxing break. But parents should assess the resources available for periodic respite. Respite is a term meaning a relief period. The length of respite can be a few minutes to several days or weeks. How much respite an individual needs depends on their individual circumstances. How much respite an individual will actually get depends on many factors:

- economic status

- availability of respite and financial assistance in the area in which the family resides

- support available from friends and family (i.e. their willingness to provide respite for parents or to help them find it elsewhere)

- willingness of the parents to take the time to find respite and set it up.

Parents should assess their environment. Are there friends or extended family members who will give parents and/or their immediate family an occasional break from the more advanced child? Is there someone whom parents can afford to pay to "babysit" their child while parents get away to be alone or do things with other family members? If the parent or parents cannot afford to pay for respite services, check with the appropriate department or ministry (e.g., department of mental health, developmental services, mental retardation, etc.) to determine if financial assistance is available for respite services. Is there an agency (government or private) that can help parents find and maintain respite care? Organizations in the US that can assist in locating agency/community services include:

- the family's church or synagogue

- a local chapter of the Autism Society of America

- a local chapter of the Association for Retarded Citizens

- or state or provincial agencies.

See the MAAP website (www.maapservices.org) for referrals to some of these agencies.

Even if parents haven't yet felt a desperate need for respite yet, it would be wise to locate a source of respite before the need becomes great. *The times when parents will need respite the most will be when they are feeling too tired to look for it.*

MAKE A DIRECTORY AND GUIDE FOR THOSE WHO MAY HAVE TO HELP YOUR OFFSPRING WHEN YOU CANNOT BE THERE

Please see below for an example:

Autism Directory of Services	
Name: Phone: Address: Height: Weight: Date of birth:	[Attach photo here]
Parent's name: Phone: Email: Address:	

Where child received diagnosis: Diagnosing doctor: Phone number: Address:	
Name of pediatrician or physician: Phone number: Address:	
Current medications	
Name of medication:	Daily Dosage:
Name of medication:	Daily Dosage:
Name of medication:	Daily Dosage:
Allergies:	
Name of dentist: Phone number: Address:	
Name of eye doctor: Phone number: Address:	
Name of wrap-around agency: Phone number: Address:	
Name of private occupational therapist: Phone number: Address:	
Name of private physical therapist: Phone number: Address:	
Name of sensory integration therapist: Phone number: Address:	

Summer camps and other places of recreation: Phone numbers:
Other therapists (in-home or private): Name: Phone number: Address:
Educational attorney's name: Phone number: Address:
Family attorney's name (deals with autism issues): Phone number: Address:
Child's educational advocate: Phone number: Address:
Child's school name: Phone number: Address:
Residential placement (present and/or past): Phone number: Address:
Other organizations that have been useful to you (services they provide and phone numbers):
Extended family member's name: Relationship to person: Phone number: Address:

Paid support individuals (include rate of pay and average hours per week or month): Peer mentors: Housekeeper: Bookkeeper: Other helpers:
Person's likes and dislikes:

Recommendations for Late Teens and Adults

In an adult, finding a diagnosis may be very helpful in determining the job and community supports that are needed. Also, having a name for what makes one feel different or presents challenges in everyday life can be a great relief to an adult. Many have shared that they used to think they were just "strange" or a "failure." Once they received a diagnosis, they understood that many of their life barriers were due to an ASD.

Most late teens and adults begin to suspect they have some form of autism, and then seek out information and resources to confirm or deny their suspicions. In other cases, parents, close friends, employers, or teachers begin to suspect this may be the case. Here are general recommendations for those who suspect some form of ASD.

READING

If you think you may be on the autism spectrum, try reading books written by other individuals on the autism spectrum and see if things in their life ring true for you. Here is just a partial list of such books:

- *Asperger's From the Inside Out* by Michael John Carley
- *Pretending to Be Normal* by Liane Holliday Willey

- *Beyond the Wall* by Stephen Shore
- *Emergence: Labeled Autistic* by Temple Grandin
- *Your Life is Not a Label* by Jerry Newport
- *A Real Person* by Gunilla Gerlund
- *Look Me In the Eye* by John Elder Robinson
- *Build Your Own Life* by Wendy Lawson
- *Middle School: The Stuff Nobody Tells You* by Haley Moss (for teen girls).

SEEK A DIAGNOSIS

Be sure that the place from which you seek the diagnosis has experience with *more cognitively advanced people* who are 15 years and older. By now, you may have learned to cope with your differences to such an extent that they will no longer be evident to the inexperienced observer. Presentation of symptoms in older teens and adults are often quite different from those of children. Also, those who have only seen younger and more severe individuals often miss the more subtle symptoms you may now present. Your parents, an older relative who knows you well, or a close friend who has known you for many years would be a great help to someone attempting an accurate diagnosis.

JOIN VIRTUAL AND/OR IN-PERSON GROUPS OF INDIVIDUALS WITH AUTISM OR ASPERGER SYNDROME

Many of these groups refer to themselves as "Aspies." The majority prefers the Asperger syndrome classification to that of autism because of a history of the general public regarding autism as a more severe condition, in terms of cognitive and social abilities. Although there are many brilliant and accomplished people with autism, the public perception tends to remain. Here is a very small list of such groups:

- GRASP (www.grasp.org)
- AGUA (myweb.lmu.edu/jdevine/AS/AGUA_Classic.mht)
- OASIS @ MAAP community forums (www.asperger syndrome.org)
- Asperger Employment Issues (Google Chat Group, www. google.com)

The place or person who gives you a diagnosis may know of local groups.

DISCLOSURE

Contemplate the issue of disclosure in both your personal, academic, and professional life. There is no one decision for all. Many books are written about this including:

- *Asperger's From the Inside Out* by Michael John Carley
- *Beyond the Wall* by Stephen Shore
- *Developing Talents* by Temple Grandin and Kate Duffy

SUPPORT

With the help of trusted friends and mentors, investigate whether or not you qualify for any government help. This will depend on your country of citizenship, your employment potential and your ability to live on your own. If you need help or guidance in finding these forms of support, contact any national advocacy group your country has that deals with autism.

REHEARSE VARIOUS SITUATIONS

Go over "scripts" with mentors that detail what information you need to share and what questions you need to ask when approaching:

- medical help
- diagnosis
- education
- employment
- (in some cases) human services and advocacy groups.

This is because it is often hard for people within the autism spectrum to know what is the most important information for a non-spectrum person to process in order to be effective. It is like asking where the bathroom is in English when you are in a French-speaking country. You must translate your information and the length thereof into "non-spectrumese." Some people actually use lists or cue cards and tick them off as they present the information.

When we non-spectrum people get too much or incomplete (by our standards) information, we may fail to help you due to misunderstanding your needs or due to shutting off our processing at some point.

I realize fully that the same is true when people not on the autism spectrum need to tell you their needs or questions!

Chapter 4

The ASD Adult at Home

The advice in the previous chapter applies to parents of both young and adult offspring. However, there are some considerations that are particularly important to those parents who have an adult with an ASD.

Parents of adults should—if they have not already done so—seek legal advice about how they may best plan for their challenged loved one's financial and other needs for that time when parents are no longer around to attend to those needs. In the case of highly advanced individuals, a special needs trust may not be appropriate—especially if they have an above-minimum-wage job. In some of those cases limited guardianships can help. In addition, parents of challenged adults must realize that when they die, their child will still need someone to serve as an advocate on an ongoing basis. It is very important to cover the legal planning, guardianships and wills with legal professionals experienced in developmental disabilities law.

Counting on siblings to fulfill this duty may seem simple, but what if the other children move far away? What if they marry someone who does not want them to assume that responsibility? What if the neuro-typical child predeceases the child with autism? Back-up provisions should be made. Each parent must assess their challenged offspring and the environment in which they wish him to live and then determine what arrangements they can make to facilitate a secure and successful future for him.

Parents should assess possible candidates for full or partial guardianship. Perhaps a local agency supports a group home or semi-independent apartment arrangement in which he can live. If he is capable of living on his own, perhaps that agency can be the one who checks on him at regular intervals and acts as his advocate. Parents must be very realistic about what they can expect from their more advanced loved one and what they can expect from others. Parents should make the best decisions possible. Then the parent or parents must realize that their challenged loved one is probably better off adjusting to this ultimate environment *before* they die. The death of a parent or both parents will be a difficult adjustment for him. Trying to adjust to a new living environment at the same time could be devastating for him.

I believe, as both a parent and a long-time advocate for people with autism, that the interests of the more advanced adult are best met when she does not reside with her parents as an adult. This enables parents to properly set up and supervise her ultimate living environment for a longer period of time. Certainly, this is an extremely difficult issue. However, for the sake of the loved one with any ASD, this issue must be faced.

Chapter 5

Schooling for the ASD Individual

Selecting a School and Classroom Setting

All I can do here is speak in generalities, because the ideal school and classroom placement for each individual will vary according to age, level of academic achievement, behavior strengths and difficulties, and estimated potential academic ability (see Appendix C). In addition, placement options depend on the proximity of the school to the parents and the economic resources available to that family. For example, there may be a terrific Montessori school nearby which fits a child's needs perfectly. However, the school system may not pay expenses at the Montessori school, and the tuition may be unaffordable for some families. Or, that Montessori school may be 90 minutes from the family's home. In reality, the ease and speed of placement depends on the philosophy of the school district and availability of programming.

Regardless of the functioning level of the child, each individual family must evaluate whether to pursue education at a day school or residential setting. This is a difficult and agonizing decision that cannot be judged for others. Ideally, parents should consider the welfare of other siblings and their own ability to carry through consistently with behavioral approaches in the home setting. Trusted experts, other family members, and the parent's own mind and heart must be consulted before this decision is made. Remember, parents are the primary decision-maker and advocate for their child with a disability. The final placement determination, however, must be made through the annual case conference and is based on the recommendations of the multidisciplinary team.

In their attempts to procure teachers who know about ASDs and who are trained in current teaching techniques that are most effective for ASD children, many parents and professionals have insisted on segregated classrooms. In most cases, the least desirable placement for an ASD student is a setting that contains exclusively peers with social disabilities. The ASD student needs and often wants interaction with non-disabled peers or socially average disabled peers. Role models for *positive* peer interaction can be better provided by neuro-typical peers, as well as peers with challenges that do not affect the ability to interact socially (e.g., Down syndrome). Conversely, a placement with children who experience similar handicapping conditions promotes an environment that maintains similarities across students. For example, placing students together who experience aggressive behavior will establish a setting that may increase the occurrence of this problem behavior. Obviously, this type of placement is not desirable. Therefore, a more typical education setting is preferable if all other considerations are equal. Parents should observe the overall atmosphere of the school. Is the school run in a reasonably orderly fashion? Is the climate a positive one? What is the attitude of the principal of the school about accommodating someone with different needs? Are classroom sizes relatively small?

The probable classroom and teacher placement for the child must be ascertained. Is the climate of the classroom organized and reasonably quiet? Is the teacher positive, creative, flexible, and consistent? Can appropriately trained personnel be available to provide special services? Is the classroom arranged to accommodate peer instruction and cooperative learning?

Placement of these unique children involves making difficult decisions. Both parents and guiding professionals may fear making a less than ideal choice. About the best one can do is evaluate the choices carefully and then follow through with a positive feeling of commitment.

Preparing the Child for School Placement

There are many things that parents can do to prepare their ASD child for a successful school experience. First and most important, is to instill a positive attitude in the child. The term "positive" has been used a great deal in this book. It can *never* be used enough! A negative attitude by a professional or the parent can be communicated to the child by word, deed, or attitude. This negative attitude becomes the catalyst to a downward spiral of events and attitudes that promotes failure for the ASD student. Always investigate your concerns about the child and his services, but confine your inquiries to the appropriate people. The ASD student has enough problems getting through each day. Don't add doubt and fear to his list of woes by displaying negative actions and attitudes.

An example of the effect of negative parental attitude can be shown in the case of a parent who engaged me as her son's advocate. The parent felt that her son's teacher had a negative attitude toward her son. According to the parent, her son was increasingly resisting going to school. Upon talking with all concerned parties, I found out that the teacher did indeed have a negative attitude, which was easily rectified upon being properly informed about ASDs. However, I also found out that the parent was sending the child off to school each day, saying, "I hope you'll be O.K. at school today. I hope the teacher won't be too mean to you." No wonder the child didn't want to go to school!

The ASD student often has trouble with time concepts, especially involving a schedule. Provide her with information about what time she will go to the new school. Then explain at what time she will leave school and when she will arrive home. If she doesn't know how to tell time using a watch, explain her daily schedule in reference to other milestones she *does* understand. For example, "You will leave the house for school after you have eaten breakfast and brushed your teeth. You will get on the bus to leave school after you have finished your music class, put your books away at your desk, and gotten your coat out of your locker." A calendar, a written or picture schedule, or a diagram depicting the student walking through the different stages of the school day will assist her in understanding and being comfortable with her daily schedule.

Teach the child how to navigate her school. This can be done by showing her a detailed map of the school and then tracing her path through the school from the beginning of her day to the end, or by actually walking her through the school, simulating her school day from beginning to end. Sometimes combining both of these strategies is necessary. In other instances, ongoing training and/or support by the teacher, an aide, or a peer tutor may be necessary until she learns the pattern of her movements. In all cases, when the order of her movement from place to place is going to be altered (such as on Monday after lunch there is no gym), you will need to tell her ahead of time to prepare her properly. As these children get older, most of them greatly increase their ability to navigate, and their flexibility in handling changes in routine. However, in the first schooling experience, explaining and demonstrating where to go and preparing her for changes in her routine are almost always necessary. Sometimes ASD people need training and support well into adulthood whenever their environment changes significantly. Others are very skilled in moving from place to place, but remain unskilled in knowing *when* to go *where*.

Many need to be shown a "safe place" and/or a "safe person" they can go to when confused or upset during their school day. This gives them the feeling of control, which most of us need. The "safe place" could be the school office, a counselor's office, or any place where he can get away from classmates and the classroom or whatever environment upset him. The setting should be calm and quiet. The "safe person" can be a school nurse, the school principal, or a counselor. The main requirement for the "safe person" is that he has a good understanding of the child's specific problems and demonstrates a kind and empathic manner. For some children, just giving them a hall pass and providing them the option to leave or go to the bathroom for a few minutes will be sufficient. ASD students who have been provided this option seldom, if ever, abuse it. For the most part, they dislike change in their routine, even if the change is an enjoyable activity. Leaving the classroom to go to the office or other safe place is most often perceived as a change in routine.

Before the ASD child begins his schooling a person should be designated to act as a liaison between him and those with whom he comes in contact during his school day, including the bus driver, librarian, principal, music teacher, gym teacher, and playground supervisor. The liaison should assist staff to facilitate a smooth transition from one grade and school to another. This liaison should also act as a liaison between home and school and must recognize the need for frequent information exchange between parents and teachers. The liaison could be the school psychologist, school counselor, teacher, or any interested professional. In the majority of real-life situations, the only knowledgeable liaison for the child is the parent. This is certainly not the way things should be, but lack of knowledge about the needs of ASD individuals, combined with the rapid turnover of staff assigned to help the individual and his family, usually necessitate parents' participation in this role.

Preparation for Teaching the More Advanced Student

Teachers working with ASD students for the first time will need training. This includes both general teachers and special educators alike. Teachers who have the greatest misconceptions about the more advanced ASD child have had previous experience teaching other ASD children who are less advanced.

Some professionals find it hard to accept that these children, whose symptoms appear to be less severe, are in fact challenged by the same disabilities as other individuals within the autism spectrum. They read the behavior as deliberate and obstinate, rather than a different manifestation of ASDs.

Recognizing important characteristics of ASD students will aid the teacher's efforts. Chapter 6 lists some basic tips for teachers. They were originally developed by Carol O'Neal of School District #52 in Darien, Illinois. I then added a few and elaborated others.

Chapter 6

Tips for Teaching and Students

1. Many ASD people have trouble with *organizational skills*, regardless of their intelligence and/or age. Others are extremely organized, even to the point of being obsessive. A "straight A" student with a photographic memory can be incapable of remembering to bring a pencil to class or remembering a deadline for an assignment. In such cases, aid should be provided in the least restrictive way possible. Strategies could include having the child put a picture of a pencil on the cover of his notebook or written reminders at the end of the day of assignments to be completed at home. Always praise the child when he remembers something he has previously forgotten. Never scold or "harp" at him when he fails. A lecture on the subject will not only *not* help, it will often make the problem worse. He may begin to believe he *can't* remember to do or bring these things.

   These students seem to have either the neatest or the messiest desks or lockers in the school. The one with the neatest desk or locker is probably very insistent on sameness and will be very upset if someone disturbs the order she has created. The one with the messiest desk will need your help in frequent cleanups of the desk or locker so that she may find things. Simply remember that the student is probably not making a conscious choice to be messy, she is most likely incapable of this organization task without specific training. Train her in organizational skills using small, specific steps.

2. ASD students often have *problems with abstract and conceptual thinking.* Some may eventually acquire a few abstract skills, but others never will. Avoid abstract ideas when possible. When abstract concepts must be used, use visual cues, such as gestures, or written words to augment the abstract idea.

3. An *increase in unusual or difficult behaviors usually indicates an increase in stress.* Sometimes stress is caused by feeling a loss of control. When this occurs, the "safe place" or "safe person" may come in handy, because *many* times the stress will only be alleviated when the student physically removes himself from the stressful event or situation. If this occurs, a program should be set up to assist the student in re-entering and/or staying in the stressful situation.

4. *Don't take misbehaviors personally.* The ASD student is not a manipulative, scheming person who is trying to make life difficult. Usually misbehavior is the result of efforts to survive experiences that may be confusing, disorienting, or frightening. People with ASDs are, by virtue of their handicap, egocentric and have extreme difficulty reading the reactions of others. They are largely incapable of being manipulative.

5. Most ASD students *use and interpret speech literally.* Until you know the capabilities of the individual, you should avoid:

   ○ idioms ("save your breath," "jump the gun," "second thoughts," etc.)

   ○ double meanings (most jokes have double meanings)

   ○ sarcasm (such as saying, "Great!" after he has just spilled a bottle of ketchup on the table)

- nicknames

- "cute" names, such as Pal, Buddy, Wise Guy, etc.

6. Be *as concrete as possible* in all your interactions with these students. Remember that facial expression and other social cues may not work. Avoid asking questions such as, "Why did you do that?" Instead, say, "I didn't like the way you slammed your book down on the desk and got up to leave for the gym." In answering essay questions that require a synthesis of information, ASD individuals rarely know when they have said enough or if they are properly addressing the core of the question.

7. If the student doesn't seem to be able to learn a task, *break it down into smaller steps* or present the task in several different ways (e.g., visually, verbally, physically).

8. Avoid *verbal overload*. Be clear. Use shorter sentences if you perceive that the student doesn't fully understand you. Although he probably has no hearing problem and may be paying attention, he may have a problem understanding your main point and identifying the most important information.

9. *Prepare the student for all environmental and/or routine changes*, such as assembly, substitute teacher, rescheduling, etc. Use her written or visual schedule to prepare her for change.

10. Behavioral supports work, but if incorrectly used, they can encourage robot-like behavior, provide only a short-term behavior change, or result in aggression. Use *positive* and chronologically age-appropriate procedures.

11. Consistent *treatment* and expectations from *everyone* is vital.

12. Be aware that normal *levels of auditory and visual input* can be perceived by the student as too much or too little. For example, the hum of fluorescent lighting

is extremely distracting for some people with ASDs. Consider environmental changes such as removing some of the "visual clutter" from the room or seating changes if the student seems distracted or upset by his classroom environment.

13. If the ASD student uses *repetitive verbal arguments* and/or repetitive verbal questions, try requesting that he write down the question or argumentative statement. Then write down your reply. As the writing continues, the more advanced student usually begins to calm down and stop the repetitive activity. If that doesn't work, write down his repetitive verbal question or argument, and then ask him to formulate and write down a logical reply or a reply he thinks you would make. This distracts the student from escalating the verbal aspect of the argument or question and sometimes provides a more socially acceptable way of expressing frustration or anxiety.

If the student does not read or write, try role-playing the repetitive verbal question or argument with the teacher taking the student's part and the student answering the teacher. Continually responding in a logical manner or arguing back seldom stops this behavior. The subject of their argument or question is not always the subject that has upset the student. The argument or question more often communicates a feeling of loss of control or uncertainty about someone or something in the environment.

ASD individuals often have trouble "getting" your points. If the repetitive verbal argument or question persists, consider the possibility that she is very concerned about the topic and does not know how to rephrase the question or comment to get the information she needs.

14. ASD individuals experience various communication difficulties. Unless it is tried on an experimental basis with follow-up, or unless the teacher is already *certain*

that the student has mastered this skill, *don't rely on the ASD student to relay important messages* to their parents about school events, assignments, school rules, etc. Sending home a note for his parents may not even work. The student may not remember to deliver the note or may lose it before reaching home. Phone calls to the parent work best until this skill can be developed. Frequent and accurate communication between the teacher and parent (or primary caregiver) is very important.

15. If a classroom activity involves *pairing off* or choosing partners, either draw numbers or use some other arbitrary means of pairing. Or ask an especially kind student if he would agree to choose the ASD individual as a partner. This should be arranged before the pairing is done. The ASD student is most often the individual left with no partner. This is unfortunate since these students could benefit most from having a partner.

Additional Tips

In the classroom it is very easy to misunderstand the actions and reactions of ASD individuals. Margaret Dewey (Dewey and Everard, 1974), an author and parent of an adult with autism, says there are three pieces of simplistic advice often given to ASD students by their teachers, which are erroneous and ineffective. Remember them and *avoid them when dealing with anyone within the advanced spectrum of disorders.*

1. "Try to learn from listening," or "You're not listening." Sometimes a teacher has given a stream of instructions which the person with ASD has difficulty in prioritizing and acting upon. At other times, he is not able to determine exactly what the teacher thought was important. In either case, too often the [ASD] person thinks she is doing what she is supposed to be doing, when suddenly the

teachers says to her, "That's the last straw. If you can't pay attention you'll have to leave the room."

2. "Just take it easy. Stop being so tense. Everything will be O.K." [ASD] people are often tense and for good reason. They know from experience that things can go wrong unexpectedly. Few supposedly normal people can relax upon command, so why expect an ASD person to be able to do so? Instead of telling them to take it easy, redirect them or move them into a different environment temporarily if possible. This may help relieve the stressful situation. (It might be helpful to teach them a relaxation response to use in very tense situations.)

3. "Stop being so self-centered." Of course an ASD person seems self-centered. Her viewpoint is the only one which is clear to her.

Dewey's point about teachers thinking that the ASD student isn't listening becomes critical in situations where test instructions are given. Not only may the student not understand the important points in the instructions, *they will almost never tell the teacher they don't understand.*

Most important, if teachers treat these students with an open mind and a positive attitude, it can be a very rewarding experience. Individuals with ASDs have tremendous potential. Teachers can be instrumental in helping them achieve that potential!

Preparing Fellow Students

Just as the ASD student and his teachers must be properly prepared for the schooling experience, fellow students should be prepared as well. Classroom peers should be told about the ASD student and how they can be of help to him. Most children tease their disabled peers when they fear or misunderstand his actions or motivations, or when they simply don't believe that the peer is, indeed, disabled.

An excellent way to help fellow students understand the sensory perception problems of the ASD student is to use the hypothetical simulation of the experience of distorted sensory information. I have used this approach with both students and teachers for several years. Usually the students or teachers end up jumping up out of their seats, pulling away, or acting startled in some other way. The simulation helps them achieve an empathic understanding that the reasons for some supposedly illogical behaviors are, in fact, quite logical if you are experiencing a situation with sensory processing problems. A full description of this simulation follows in the next chapter.

Chapter 7

Sensory Distortion Simulation

Approximate Time (per demonstration)

15 to 20 minutes

Description

This simulation (done by three presenters) is intended to be a participatory demonstration of the experience of receiving confusing and/or distorted sensory information. The intent of this experience is to demonstrate to typical people what the sensory difficulties of the more advanced student with autism or Asperger syndrome may be like.

Required Area and Equipment

- A relatively small room that can be darkened easily.

- Enough chairs and desks for the participants.

- At least two electrical outlets.

- One presenter needs access to a light switch to control lighting in the room.

- Pencils and papers for all participants.

- Two radios and extension cords.

- Two special gloves (one cotton exfoliating bath glove and one very damp cotton glove).

- Three or four handkerchiefs soaked in a strong perfume or two differently scented room sprays.

- Two heavy books.

- Inflated balloons and a pin to pop them.

- One central presenter and two aides.

Demonstration

Start the demonstration by explaining to the students that you are going to give them an experience that can help them to understand how hard it can be for a student with an ASD—or with attention deficit disorder (ADD) and some other learning challenges—to sit still and do what is asked of them in class, due to the many sensory challenges they may face that we don't. Explain that everything from smells coming from the cafeteria or other "smelly" things in school like paint or glue or even strong perfumes and aftershaves, to the humming of the fluorescent lighting in the classroom, to people talking or walking in the halls, to unexpected loudspeaker announcements, to slamming lockers and closing doors, can create sensory shocks that may disturb them, but that we supposedly more typical people barely notice. Tell them to imagine they're a new student with a disability in a new classroom. All they want to do is fit in and get through the day.

1. Participants are instructed to find a chair and told that they are in their new classroom.

   ○ "Teacher" introduces him/herself and says that participants must only follow a few simple rules to get along happily in their new classroom: sit still in their seats, follow simple directions, and be reasonably quiet.

- The teacher says students will be given a short spelling test consisting of words that are below the grade level of the students in the room.

2. Simulations occur simultaneously to distort the senses of the participants.

   - The teacher begins the spelling test as she walks around the room near the students, talking alternately too loud and too soft, and using a distorted manner of speech.

   - The teacher pats the students' hands and faces (in mock consolation) with the special gloves, alternating the rough glove on one student and the wet one on the next student.

   - Lights can be dimmed and brightened or turned on and off *slowly*. The slow pace of this is essential to prevent causing a student with seizure disorder from any problems.

   - The radio is turned on loud at a point between radio stations, so that loud "white noise" is created.

   - The teacher and aides wave handkerchiefs soaked in strong perfume or spray two different scents of room spray alternately. (Don't make it too heavy or people might cough or sneeze—this is a distortion, not torture!)

   - Aides drop heavy books and pop balloons at irregular intervals.

   All of the above "testing" activities take place simultaneously.

3. The teacher reacts to the students' negative reactions to above distractions.

   - When participants pull back and begin to make a noise, the teacher claps her hands, stamps her foot, and shouts "Stop!" simultaneously.

- ◦ At *exactly that same time* all of the sights and sounds of the simulation cease, and the lights are turned back on.
- ◦ The teacher says in a firm and unhappy voice, "Let me see your tests." She notes out loud that few students have written very many of the "spelling words."
- ◦ The teacher says, "If you can't pay attention and try in my class, you are out of here!"

4. Discussion: The teacher then asks the students if they think they would be in trouble if they acted like they did in the simulation during regular class time. What would happen to their grades if they regularly performed like this on tests?

Discussion then follows between the presenters and the participants about how this simulation attempts to approximate the sensory experiences of more advanced students with autism, Asperger syndrome, or pervasive developmental disorder—not otherwise specified, and how those sensory processing problems can be mistaken for deliberate misbehavior and restlessness.

A very creative parent I met used this simulation and added a great feature to it. After the simulation, while they were talking things over, she gave each student a Tootsie Pop. The students then could eat the Tootsies while listening and talking. Near the end of the discussion, she would then say, "Is this Tootsie Pop the same on the inside as it is on the outside? When the students reply, "No," she says that most people are like that and that ASD students or any student who copes with some challenge in life can be like that too.

Caution: People who have any reason to suspect they are prone to seizures should *not* be exposed to the flickering lights, as this may trigger seizure activity.

Chapter 8

Older Teen and Young Adult Students with ASDs

Decisions About Where to Live, Further Education, and Training

As ASD individuals leave high school, they must decide about career pathways and living options that are available to them. This is usually done in consultation with caregivers and trusted mentors. Do they want to go into a trade school, an apprenticeship, a junior college, a community college, or a traditional college or university? Do they want, and can they economically afford, to take a break for a few months or weeks? Do they want to live at home or on their own or in an optional communal setting (group home, supervised apartment, religious setting)?

These are huge and important decisions. Often even the parents and mentors are not sure which options are best. The best approach is to get as much input as possible. Parents need to help compile this information (preferably in writing) and then present it in segments to the teen or adult. This process is sometimes made easier by the determination and opinions of the ASD individual. My daughter was determined to attend college since her freshman year in high school. She wanted to live away from home, both in college and after college. The prospect terrified me, as her parent, when she announced all this to me at age 16. I truly didn't think she had the skills to live away from us yet, though we were working hard on that and had been since she was in grade school. I just didn't know if she had the skills to do it, but I knew she had the courage. She proved us wrong and went on to live at college, graduate in four years and continue on through graduate school. This was made possible by hard work, careful planning, her skill and determination, and a great deal of plain luck.

In other cases, individuals may want to attain a college degree for the sake of securing a good job or for the fulfillment of their quest for higher knowledge about an area of academic interest. Others may seek an apprenticeship, or trade school, or junior college for the same reasons. Many choose to attend one of these options within their current community for the sake of familiarity and the ability to stay at home. I might add that in the United States, many non-spectrum teens are making the latter choice for the same reasons.

Since one of the goals of this book is not to be too lengthy, I will address choosing a college.

How to Select a College and Prepare for Your College Experience

Selecting a College

SOME QUESTIONS TO ASK YOURSELF

- What do you expect to accomplish in your time at college?

- Are you comfortable with the idea of trying to live at the college, or should you look at community college options within a reasonable commute from home?

- Do you want a private, double or quad room? This is a good issue to assess with your parents and trusted mentors.

- Do you want to attend a small college or a larger one?

  Advantages of small colleges:

  ○ More personal attention.

  ○ Not easy to get "lost in the crowd."

  ○ Sometimes easier to access help for problems with a difficult class or a personal problem.

  Disadvantages of small colleges:

  ○ Sometimes small colleges are more expensive.

  ○ Smaller colleges have fewer course options.

  ○ Due to fewer students, your "mistakes" may be noticed more easily.

  Advantages of large colleges:

  ○ More course options.

  ○ More sports opportunities and activities clubs.

  ○ You can be more anonymous, both in class and socially.

  Disadvantages of large colleges:

  ○ It is harder to get personal attention from your professors at a larger college.

  ○ There is a greater probability of getting "lost in the crowd."

  ○ It is sometimes harder to make friends in a larger number of people.

- ○ Physically navigating a larger college might be difficult.

QUESTIONS TO ASK A PROSPECTIVE COLLEGE

- What are your minimum scholastic requirements?
- Do you offer any scholarships that might pertain to me?
- Do you have an office of special services? Have they been successful in accommodating other students like me?
- Do you have free scholastic tutoring available?
- Do incoming freshmen have student and/or faculty mentors?
- If I need a private room, can I get one as a freshman? How much more does this cost?

THINGS TO OBSERVE DURING CAMPUS VISITS

- Are the students friendly?
- Is the person you deal with in the office of special services friendly and interested in you?
- Is the person in charge of student affairs friendly and easily accessible?
- Are there lots of things to do on campus?
- Are there exercise facilities?
- Is there a swimming pool?
- Are there tennis courts?
- Are there good walking or jogging areas?
- Is the campus near town?
- Are stores going to be easy for you to access?

- Are the dorms convenient and what you had hoped for? Are they air conditioned?

The rest is entirely a personal decision. Go where you feel welcomed and most comfortable. Go where you think you will accomplish the most items included in your personal success goals.

When my daughter chose a smaller campus, she based her decision on several things:

- she was accepted academically, despite SAT scores

- they had the course of study she wanted

- the students were friendly, as was the administration

- she already knew someone she liked and trusted on the campus.

Preparing Yourself for the College Experience

- Attend at least one "prospective students' day" at any college you are considering (as well as an appointment-based interview visit).

- Attend a prospective students' weekend, if possible. If you need someone to accompany you (out of necessity or just out of comfort), you may request this with the special services department. *This is another thing to talk to your parents and/or trusted mentors about.*

- Before your first semester, learn where things are on the campus, through studying campus maps and from visits to the college.

- Learn what the students on campus wear, typically, to class (by season).

- Check with your parents, the college's office of special services, and trusted mentors about where you can seek help for:
  - getting academic help in a subject
  - learning about campus activities
  - resolving conflicts with fellow students.
- Get a copy of the student handbook and begin to learn what is in it (school rules, grading periods and policies, vacation schedule, etc.).

Some Adjustments You May Need

- Extra time in taking tests.
- Notes and/or outlines written for you by a fellow student or provided by the professor.
- Tutors in various subjects.
- Peer mentor.
- Faculty mentor.
- Tell Special Services that you need to be notified as soon as any professor thinks your grades and/or study habits are declining.

This workbook is highly recommended: *The College Companion: Your Survival Guide to College Life* by Susan Orenstein, www.orensteinsolutions.com.

Chapter 9

Individuals with ASD in the Community

For an ASD individual to enjoy a full life, he must be able to access community resources. Ventures into the community can include shopping, working, getting haircuts, eating at fast food restaurants, and participating socially. To facilitate a more enjoyable and successful experience, he must be properly prepared.

Some parents and/or teachers feel that the probability of a successful community experience is enhanced by providing basic information about the ASD individual to key people, including the local grocer, librarian, or police personnel. Others feel that sharing information is seldom or never necessary. In my experience, it helps if community members understand the potential problems these individuals have in interpreting social situations. This can be presented in a casual manner without causing undue embarrassment, and preserving the dignity of the challenged person. However, be careful and cognizant of being sure that the ASD individual for whom you are attempting this agrees with the idea of disclosure to these key people in the community.

Informing the local police department about the special problems that may result from having an ASD person residing in the community is an issue that is unpleasant for parents. Unfortunately, incidents resulting from uninformed police misinterpreting the actions of ASD people have provided a convincing argument for the dissemination of information.

Several years ago a teenager with autism was arrested for failing to notice pretty girls on the beach. The girls thought he must be "on drugs" and reported him to the police. Another young man was arrested for failing to follow a policeman's verbal directions in a parking lot. A third man was near the scene of a crime. He was innocent, but failed to stop when ordered to by police because his mother had instructed him not to stop on the way home or talk to strangers. At the door of his house, the police caught him and handled him so roughly he had permanent kidney damage. Although these individuals were cleared of all charges, the experiences were traumatic. The issue of talking to police is serious business! However, ASD does *not* cause intentional criminal behavior.

When contacting local police about your challenged child or adult, be sure they receive a recent photograph and a written physical description. When you speak with someone in the police department, make sure that information will be disseminated to other police officers. Don't just tell them that this person is challenged. Explain problems such as aggressive behavior, repetitive verbal arguments, avoiding strangers by running away from them, lack of understanding of social convention, or ability to get lost easily. In addition, it should be explained that if these individuals are questioned under what they perceive to be a pressure situation, they will answer with what they think the interrogator wants to hear, or will just keep answering "yes." If the police are ever involved in an incident with the individual in the community, they will understand why the individual may be behaving in an unusual or antisocial way. Their understanding could help in averting unnecessary arrest and/or restraint by police. In addition, these law enforcement personnel may be able to help if the challenged person is missing. It is generally agreed that firemen and local hospital emergency room personnel should also be informed about the challenged person.

Obviously the employer of an ASD individual should be given all relevant information. More advanced individuals often make wonderful and dependable employees. They are usually consistent in speed and quality of job performance. Their insistence on sameness and routine make most of them very punctual. Many have high-level vocational skills. Some need limited hours and the flexibility to leave the workplace if they are overwrought. Successful job placement may be facilitated by seeking jobs that allow the individual to pursue her peak skill or interest area, while taking into consideration individual socialization or work access problems. Employment situations are most successful when a liaison is available to assist the challenged person and her employer. This liaison can help with any behavior problems and speak on behalf of the individual when she has a work grievance.

Unfortunately, work opportunities are still very few for ASD adults. What we most often find is that these adults often have high intelligence and can be trained in what should be high-paying jobs, but are not given employment in those careers after training. Instead, they are offered jobs that are drastically below skill level. In addition, the state Department of Vocational Rehabilitation system that is supposed to provide job training and placement services for these individuals in the United States is grossly inept at dealing with ASD individuals. When it even allows them services, it misunderstands both their needs and talents. The following letter from Volume 1 of the 1998 *The MAAP Newsletter* is an excellent illustration of this situation.

> I am a 38-year-old man with autism. I grew up in an era (60s and 70s) before IEPs [individualized education programs] or special education classes. I was mainstreamed [see Glossary] before the hot shots invented the word, as public school was the only thing available, and believe me it was tough. Yes, Vocational Rehabilitation needs improvement and a great deal of reform. It is designed for either [physically disabled] people or severely mentally retarded people. To them autism is still hopeless and to want to have a job above janitor or sheltered workshop

or anything that's low skill and low pay with no future is considered unrealistic goals. My mom and I quit dealing with them, as it was a waste of time. To get into Voc Rehab one has to hop through too many hoops to satisfy the bureaucracy and for nothing!! It's too easy for some VR [Vocational Rehabilitation] Counselor to sit in his chair in his office and say "unrealistic goals" and "we will let you be a janitor." Or they put you through training for a job and then won't help you get a job.

In my case, it was for Pharmacy Technician. With VR they put me through the training, set up the student loan, and when I finished the training with an A+ average, VR refused to help me get a job in a pharmacy in a hospital. They brought up "liability." What liability? The liability that I would do well? That I take the time to do a job right?

The big problem is that I worked to be a Pharmacy Tech. I repaid the loan for $3500 and never got to use the training. I have worked in the Central Service [supply department] but because of attitudes, I got fired. I since moved back to Kansas City, MO, and after three plus years of unemployment am back in Central Service of a local hospital. (Wade, 1998)

Whether or not others in the community should be informed depends on individual and family preferences. Some people feel that preparing others before meeting the individual deprives the ASD individual of his right to be judged regarding how he acts, not prejudged by how people think he will act. Others feel that providing information violates the individual's right to privacy and demonstrates a lack of respect for personal dignity. However, family preferences are affected by how well their family member with autism functions in the community and on their personal attitudes about his right to try and fail. I believe there is no clearly right or wrong decision on this subject.

It is hoped that each ASD child will be taught independent functioning skills that will help her navigate and enjoy her community from early childhood through adulthood. Ideally, appropriate community participation is taught not only by family members but also by those who provide education and support services. The very best place for the ASD person —or any individual with a disability—to learn community participation is in the community. Since ASD people may have problems generalizing information, the best place to learn how to buy groceries, for example, is in the local grocery store. Therefore, teaching grocery shopping in a mock grocery store set up in a special education classroom will not effectively teach an individual how to buy groceries in the local market. The size of the aisles, the number of items from which to select, the noise levels, the visual distractions, etc., cannot be fully and accurately simulated. She must learn in the environment in which she will live. This example holds true for all community experiences. Enroll the challenged person in as many community activities as possible. Providing an array of training opportunities is especially important for adults who have excessive leisure time and a limited selection of recreational options. Participation in church activities, YMCA sports and classes, health clubs, tennis clubs, swimming clubs, and local sporting events are a few suggestions. Chosen activities depend on the interests of the challenged individual and on the logistical problems presented in accessing these activities.

To successfully participate in the community, an ASD person must learn to:

- cross the street

- find the desired destination

- communicate any needs

- practice the social skills needed for the activity (i.e. "You don't need to talk to strangers when you go to the park, but you should say hello to people who speak to you in church, even if they are strangers")

- use available public transportation

- and, of course, learn skills needed to participate in the activity—for example, if you're going to use the local tennis club, you should either know how to play tennis or enroll in tennis lessons.

One of the greatest facilitators of independence and freedom to access the community and the world is the ability to drive. While this would be a wonderful means of access for ASD individuals, few ever get their license and some who do get a license quit driving soon after they begin. This is due to the skills needed to be a safe driver. First, one must be able to make accurate judgments about how fast to drive, how large of an interval to keep between cars, how to behave if stopped by a policeman, what to do in case of mechanical failure of the car, and what to do in case of a car accident. Some of these skills require good control of emotions and good social judgment. Both of these areas are very difficult for ASD individuals. Many of the parents who have told me that their ASD offspring drive admit that the safety of others was less of a concern at the time of the decision to get the license than the freedom of the individual. It seems wiser to encourage the use of public and other transportation alternatives when appropriate.

Navigational skills are just as important to teach in accessing community activities as they are for attending school. Some are able to participate in community activities by just being verbally briefed and then being shown a map of how to get to the activity. Most have the best chance for success when initial training is provided. Others will need careful and extensive training. Here, as in so many areas, there is a great variation in the ability and personality of the ASD individual.

At the adult level, all community skills can be taught by neuro-typical peers. At earlier age levels, many skills can be taught by peers and those that can't often still include peers in the activity. Encourage and facilitate these interactions if at all possible. These interactions are important for two reasons. First, peers can teach in a way that makes sense to the ASD individual while conveying typical attitudes and mannerisms for people of that age group. Second, loneliness and a need for peer companionship are frequent problems for the ASD teenager and adult. Time spent with the typical peer will provide the companionship wanted and needed by the ASD person.

Peers should be selected with great care. Their attitude, sincerity, and reliability are vitally important. An agreement on compensation (unless arranged through church, Scouts, or other volunteer organizations), rules followed, and days and times for meeting with the ASD person must be negotiated. Then the person must receive training about possible behaviors to expect and how the ASD person perceives the world. You must be clear and realistic about what skills to target. Typical peer companions may simply take the ASD individual to a movie, a school dance, a sporting event, or some other recreational or social activity. Peers can fill a void in the person's life that no parent or teacher can ever fill.

People with ASDs are so vulnerable to harm from people and situations that parents often wish they could keep them sheltered from the outside world. Wanting to keep a son or daughter safe from potentially traumatic and unpredictable happenings of daily life is certainly understandable. However, the quality of such a sheltered life is questionable. One of the most frightening—but often most productive—steps that parents take is allowing their ASD child the dignity of reasonable risk. Ultimately, the best way to make sure he is safe is to help him have positive relationships with as many non-disabled people as possible who are not paid to be with him.

Once parents get their challenged son or daughter "placed" in the community, whether in a group home, a supervised apartment, or in their own independent apartment or home, their worries and concerns don't magically disappear. They must help their offspring adapt to their new environment and help her work out problems that may arise. If the individual is living in her own residence, a case manager should be instrumental in assisting with these duties. However, since many of these individuals no longer qualify with US federal government criteria of "disabled," there is usually no one to help the parent with these duties. Since parents are not immortal, they must find an individual or agency that will assume these responsibilities at some point in time. Sometimes a group home or supervised apartment placement will make long-term follow-along more feasible. In other cases, the person's guardian or family members will hire a private case manager. However, this is often too expensive for most families.

I would like to remind parents and others who care that they can only do their best. There are no absolute right or wrong answers. So much depends on the personality of the ASD individual and his or her family's strength, structure, and financial situation. It is a long journey, with many travails, but tremendous rewards. I only wish I had known when my daughter was young and screaming for hours each day that we'd have the fun, *peaceful* times we now have together. I hope what I've shared with you brings families the success and joy we've known and a few less of the heartbreaks we've endured. Wherever your efforts lead you, remember the slogan with which we conclude every issue of *The MAAP Newsletter*...

You are not alone.

Glossary

Note: Other technical terms are defined in Chapter 2.

ASD or more advanced individual An individual who is challenged by autism, Asperger syndrome, or pervasive developmental disorder—not otherwise specified. The author prefers the acronym: ASDs.

Cognition Information thought processing and awareness.

DSM-IV-TR The American Psychiatric Association's *Diagnostic and Statistical Manual of Mental Disorders* (fourth edition, text revision), which is commonly accepted as the "diagnostic Bible" within the professional community. Therefore, we must contend with its boundaries, regardless of whether or not we agree with certain specifics within it.

Echolalia A type of spoken response that simply repeats a question that was asked to the speaker instead of a conventional answer, or repeated overheard dialogues, phrases, advertisements, etc.

Included The current term used instead of "mainstreamed." It means being "included" in a non-special education classroom setting.

Mainstreamed A term used mainly in the 1960s to the 1980s meaning the education of a child within his own local school and in a "regular" (non-special education) classroom.

Non-Spectrum (NS) This is a term coined by the author to refer to typical people. It is my hope that this term will replace "neuro-typical" as the latter implies a guarantee of no neurological differences. If one has cerebral palsy, they are not "neuro-typical," but they may be "non-spectrum." The same can be said with people who are plagued with migraine headaches, seizure disorders, and other neurological anomalies.

Prosody The inflection, tempo and intonation pattern of spoken words.

Appendix A

Some Advice for Others Who Care[1]

Caring friends, extended family and professionals often want to know what they should and should not do to be as helpful and supportive as possible to parents of more able people with autism. Some of the advice that I offer here pertains to parenting any challenged person. The rest is very uniquely specific to parenting a more able person with autism.

1. Do not say, "I know how you feel." No matter how close you are to the parents, no matter how many parents of challenged people you may have worked with, you still do not know how we feel. You can empathize with us, but you are not experiencing this process in our place.

2. Do try to include our loved ones with AS [autism] in your social gatherings or outings whenever appropriate. Some of my most painful memories of raising my daughter concern her being excluded from birthday and other parties of her classmates, family friends and neighbors.

3. Do not say, "You must be a very wonderful person for God to have chosen you to have this child." We parents of challenged children are no stronger, braver or purer than anyone else. I would personally lose my faith in God if I thought that God chose me or my child to bear this burden. Basically, this well-meaning statement says to us parents that you think this situation hurts and taxes us less than it would you.

1 An excerpt from: Moreno (1992) "High Level Individuals with Autism." In: G. Mesibov and E. Schopler (eds) *High-Functioning Individuals with Autism*. New York, NY: Plenum Press. Reproduced with kind permission from Springer Science+Business Media B.V.

4. Do offer us a chance for respite whenever you feel you can. Even a break of an hour can be a great help.

    When we were living in California and our daughter was two, a kind neighbor whom I barely knew called me one day when our daughter was about one and a half hours into what turned out to be a three-hour tantrum. I thought she was probably calling to complain about the noise. Instead she offered to come over and be with my daughter while I went to her house and took a swim in her pool. She explained that her teenage son had once had emotional problems, which included tantrums, so she could handle the noise and commotion. I did not take her up on her offer, but knowing that I could if necessary gave me the strength and courage to continue.

5. Do not offer unsolicited advice. We parents are often given unwanted and even stupid advice by people who think that they are experts on how to raise our children because their children are normal and ours are not. Our society imposes on parents of challenged people the terrible prejudice that they have produced damaged goods and are thus inferior people and parents.

6. Do say that you care and ask how you may be of help.

7. Do not say, "But *all* _____ (teenagers, toddlers, young men, girls, etc.) do that or have a problem with that." While it is true that what our loved ones on the AS spectrum think, feel, or have difficulties with are common to others, it is the *degree* and *extent* of the difficulty and the impact that it has on their lives and ours that is so very different.

8. If a parent seems unduly upset or discouraged over a particular problem, remember that the problem you see is not the only one the parent is dealing with. It is the reality that it is but one of the continual stream of problems.

9. When our offspring with AS is in an activity outside the home (scouting, church youth group, YMCA activity), do not assume we want to be there with them. This could be an excellent opportunity for the parent to have a break from the challenged person. I often felt that there was a sort of unspoken blackmail conveying that idea that if I wanted my challenged child in

an activity, then I must buy her way in by helping with the activity. I would not have minded if this happened with just one or two of her activities. However, this seemed to be the case in almost every activity.

10. Do not try to cheer a parent up by saying, "You don't know for sure that _____ (the challenged loved one) won't ever be able to…" We all have hopes for our children, but we work hardest to habilitate and plan for them when we are *realistic* about their probable future limitations.

11. It is all right to say, "I wish I could say something to make it better, but I don't know what that might be. I hope that the future will be good to you and your child."

12. Regressed behavior in our challenged loved ones often causes regressed behavior in parents. When a person with autism is experiencing a regression, parents experience a complete upheaval in their lives. People who have been friendly and supportive often stay away or completely sever their relationships with both the person on the spectrum and the family. Professionals often question what the parents might be doing differently at home to "cause" the regression. This is, at best, accusatory and, at worst, insulting and counter-productive.

    During the regression of their child with AS, parents become fatigued, depressed, worried to the point of panic, and more emotional than usual. This tends to shorten our patience and our tempers. Unfortunately this is the time when we need to exercise the greatest strength, patience, and logic toward our challenged child and all with whom he or she comes in contact. All friends, loved ones, and professionals should try to be extra supportive and patient during this difficult time. Times of regression are part and parcel of having an autism spectrum challenge. Seldom, if ever, can the "cause" of the regression be traced to anything that the parent is doing.

13. Parenting any person with autism, regardless of functioning level, is a very challenging experience. Do not assume that because parents have a higher-functioning person with autism, they have fewer or smaller problems. Many parents have told

me of incidents in which parents of lower-functioning people with autism have made them feel guilty about expressing their problems.

Appendix B

Advice for Medical Professionals[1]

Individuals with autism spectrum disorders (ASD) are developmentally disabled. This group includes individuals with diagnoses of autism, Asperger syndrome, and pervasive developmental disorder—not otherwise specified (PDD/NOS). They do not have a condition linked to a poor physical or social environment. Neither poor parenting nor a traumatic experience in infancy or childhood can cause an autism spectrum disorder (ASD). These individuals experience challenges in the area of communication, reciprocal social interaction, and inflexible thought processes. Their intelligence level can range from severely mentally retarded to brilliant. Some can speak fluently (although still experiencing difficulty in using speech to communicate needs, ideas, feelings, etc.) while others never produce speech. Some have very difficult behaviors, while others may simply seem mildly odd or eccentric. Some seek social contact and can even appear socially precocious, while others seem isolated and withdrawn. Most importantly, all individuals with ASD are unique personalities themselves, just like all neuro-typical individuals.

We present below some symptomatic behaviors and techniques which may prove helpful in your contact with ASD people. You will see some of these areas of challenge, while you may not see others. We hope that you will also see the vulnerability and potential of each person.

- Individuals with ASD often experience difficulties in processing sensory information. This can make them hyper or hypo sensitive to tactile, audiological or olfactory stimuli in their environment. Parents or hands-on caregivers are good sources

---

1   Susan J. Moreno, MAABS with Bruce Berget, MD.

of information about the idiosyncrasies of the individual you are treating. You can provide compassionate care by:

○ not touching the person without telling them you will do so. In some cases, you may wish to avoid touching them unless absolutely necessary. In some individuals, you may be able to touch one part of their body, but touch to another part may cause them extreme discomfort and distress. Hand touching is frequently a problem

○ not wearing strong perfumes, hairsprays, etc. when working with them. The smell of a hospital or doctor's office alone may be distressing to the individual with ASD, simply because it is so different from smells they encounter on a daily basis

○ modulating your voice to a softer level when speaking to or near them

○ keeping them away from noises such as crying babies, sirens, paging systems, monitors, etc.

○ realizing that they may not be able to tell you if something feels hot or painful.

• ASD patients experience rigidity in thought processes, which makes any and all forms of change difficult for them. This causes a need for sameness and routines. Unscheduled events, such as a medical emergency, can be extremely distressing to them. During such stressful times, they may: become inappropriately loud, use insulting language, exhibit repetitive motor activities, such as hand flapping; keep repeating the same words or phrases; or answer questions in whatever way they perceive you want them to. The latter of these behaviors can make emergency medical fact finding very difficult. Remember that obsessive-compulsive disorder is sometimes a co-occurring condition.

• Patients with ASD are frequently very literal in their interpretation of language.

○ Avoid colloquialisms such as "watch your step," "you'll catch your death of cold," and "the noise is ear-splitting."

These can be confusing and even frightening to the ASD individual.

- ○ They may refer to a headache as an "eyebrow ache."

- Both receptive and expressive language skills are usually impaired in individuals with ASD. Therefore:

    - ○ avoid verbal overload

    - ○ don't use nicknames, such as "pal," "buddy," or "little guy"

    - ○ don't tease

    - ○ be concrete in what you say. Avoid terms like "later," "just a little," or "perhaps"

    - ○ be specific in what you are asking them or what facts you want to give them.

- ASD individuals are challenged in their ability to read subtle social clues, like facial expressions and tone of voice. Be clear in stating your feelings and expectations to them. For example, if they are droning on about a subject not specific to the reason you are seeing them, instead of sighing and impatiently looking at your watch (cues we neuro-typicals often use to convey that we need to move on), say, "I need to leave in five minutes. Can we talk about your sore throat now?"

- People with ASD often have excellent memories. *Don't make promises you can't keep.*

- People with ASD are often better at visual processing than auditory processing. It may be helpful to use pictures and illustrations to make your point when explaining something to them or asking something of them.

- Time concepts are another rigid phenomenon in ASD people. *Don't make them wait.* Often the ASD person becomes so agitated when made to wait even a short time that they can't calm down for a prolonged period of time. They may even experience "flashbacks" of agitation when they return to a location where they have had to wait in the past.

- Some ASD individuals think that what they can't see doesn't exist. This can make having a large bandage or cast especially distressing. Let them *see* you cover up the affected area if this is a problem for them.

- In a small, but significant number of cases, individuals with ASD are self-abusive. This can include head-banging, finger and hand-biting, hitting their faces, etc. Those that experience this phenomenon seem unable to stop, even after severe injury has occurred. When these people are seen in a clinical setting, especially in an emergency room, they may appear to be abused by their parents or other caregivers.

- Another type of ASD individual is what we call "a runner." This means that they are compelled, at unpredictable times and places, to run away. Locked doors and windows and other safety precautions often fail to restrain them from this behavior. In an emergency room setting, you may attempt to treat these individuals and incur adamant protests from their parents about being separated from them. This is because they know only too well that the patient may escape without your notice. Problematically, often self-abusers are runners, as well. This often leads to false accusations of child abuse against the caregivers.

- People with autism are often lonely and very vulnerable people. Part of the reason for their largely misunderstood role in society is their difficulty with appropriately seeking help and being grateful for help offered and given.

- No matter how unaware an individual with ASD appears, always assume that they are processing what is being said and done around them.

Appendix C

Where in the World…? Finding the Ideal School

I am frequently approached by families that have the ability to move to any place in the United States—or in some cases anywhere in the world—in order to live in a good school district or within reasonable range of a good private program. Those families call and ask me, "Where are the best programs located?" I am sharing with you the advice I give when this question is asked of me. I am drawing not only from my own experiences with my daughter, but also with the many stories shared with me by many of you in MAAP. This is not an attempt to pontificate or discourage. It is merely an attempt to share information.

As far as I know, there is no one, ideal location or school program that can or will help all young children with autism or Asperger syndrome. A good school program would address your child as an *individual* and must learn how he best accesses information and what incentives encourage him to try harder in achieving goals. A willingness to learn about autism or already having knowledge of it certainly helps. Actually, teachers who are thoroughly knowledgeable about more severely impaired individuals with autism are sometimes not the best teachers for our more advanced offspring. They tend to think that our offspring are either not really on the autism spectrum or are not even significantly challenged.

When I first placed my daughter into a "regular" classroom, she was the first person with autism any of her teachers had ever taught. They were kind, dedicated, and flexible, so it all worked out. We each made some mistakes along the way, but we communicated openly and honestly to correct those mistakes and generate new ideas together. Things weren't always perfect, but we all gave it our best each day. However, one of her schools from those good years now has a different principal and most of her teachers have retired. I now would not recommend that particular school to one of our MAAP parents, or to parents of a child with any form of challenge.

The harsh reality is that there are no guarantees. A good program today may lose its current teachers or administration and may be a rotten program tomorrow. In addition, a teacher or school program may be perfect for my child and not good at all for yours. You need to talk to parents of children like yours, those within the same age range and areas of challenge and level of functioning. Then you need to visit a potential school. Make an appointment with the principal and find out her or his attitude and educational philosophy. Most schools eventually absorb the attitudes and personality of their administrators. Meet with potential teachers as well. You want a program staffed by positive, flexible, and creative people.

From that point on, just use your best instincts and intellect, make your choice, and approach the new environment with an attitude of expecting and giving the best, while forgiving small mistakes along the way. Communicate well and often with those who teach your child.

Most important of all, before leaving your and your child's friends, neighbors, and sometimes family behind for "greener pastures," be sure that you can't make things better where you already live.

Bibliography

American Psychiatric Association (2000) *Diagnostic and Statistical Manual of Mental Disorders (fourth edition, revised text).* Washington, D.C.: American Psychiatric Association.

Bashe, P.R. (2011) *The Parents' Guide to Teaching Kids with Asperger Syndrome and Similar ASDs.* New York, NY: Three Rivers Press.

Bashe, P.R. and Kirby, B. (2001) *The OASIS Guide to Asperger Syndrome: Advice, Support, Insight, and Inspiration.* New York, NY: Crown.

Carley, M.J. (2008) *Asperger's From the Inside Out.* New York, NY: Perigee Trade.

Coppola, M.A. (1988) "Residual Autism Newsletter." July, 2–3

Dewey, M. and Everard, M.P. (1974) "The Near-Normal Autistic Adolescent." *Journal of Autism and Childhood Schizophrenia 4,* 4, 348–356.

Donnellan, A., LaVigna, G., Negri-Shoultz, N. and Fassbender, L. (1988) *Progress Without Punishment.* New York, N.Y.: Teachers College Press.

Feinstein, A. (2010) *A History of Autism.* Chichester: Wiley-Blackwell.

Fischer, M. (1997) Letters, *The MAAP Newsletter 1,* 15–16.

Gerlund, G. (1997) *A Real Person: Life on the Outside.* London: Souvenir Press.

Grandin, T. and Duffy, K. (2004) *Developing Talents.* Shawnee Mission, KS: Autism Asperger Publishing Company.

Grandin, T. and Scariano, M. (1986) *Emergence: Labeled Autistic.* Novato, CA: Arena Press.

Holliday Willey, L. (1999) *Pretending to Be Normal.* London: Jessica Kingsley Publishers.

Lawson, W. (2003) *Build Your Own Life.* London: Jessica Kingsley Publishers.

Moss, H. (2010) *Middle School: The Stuff Nobody Tells You.* Shawnee Mission, KS: Autism Asperger Publishing.

Myles, B. and Southwick, J. (2005) *Asperger Syndrome and Difficult Moments.* Shawnee Mission, KS: Autism Asperger Publishing Company.

Newport, J. (2002) *Your Life Is Not a Label.* Arlington, TX: Future Horizons.

Newson, E. (1980) "The Socially Aware Autistic Child and Adult." Unpublished manuscript.

Newson, E., Dawson, M. and Everard, P. (1982) "The Natural History of Able Autistic People: Their Management and Functioning in Social Context." Unpublished manuscript.

Orenstein, S. *The College Companion: Your Survival Guide to College Life.* Available at www.orensteinsolutions.com/our-store.

Richards, H. (1992) Telephone conversation with Susan Moreno. January.

Sinclair, J. (1989) Letters, *The MAAP Newsletter.* Spring, 2.

Wade, S. (1998) Letters, *The MAAP Newsletter 1,* 4.

Waltz, M. (1999) *Pervasive Developmental Disorders: Finding a Diagnosis and Getting Help.* Sebastopol, CA: O'Reilly and Associates, Inc.

Index